The
ROAD **B**ACK
PROGRAM

HOW TO GET OFF
PSYCHIATRIC DRUGS SAFELY

There is Hope. There is a Solution...

2010 Edition

By JAMES HARPER N.C.

How to Get Off Psychiatric Drugs Safely 2010 Edition

ISBN-   1451513003
EAN-13 9781451513004

Patent Pending

For updates to this book, go to www.theroadback.org/updates.aspx

DEDICATION

To my mother, I thank you from the bottom of my heart. As a child you gave me a safe space to just be a child and allowed me to stumble and learn from my mistakes. As an adult you encouraged me to keep looking for new answers. With your passing this past year you have helped me learn value in each moment. Thank you and you are missed.

To my love, best friend and wife. This book would never have been written without you. This program would never have been developed without you. Your insistence in the early days is why The Road Back Program is here. Thank you.

DISCLAIMER

The claims, information and products mentioned in this book, *How to Get Off Psychiatric Drugs Safely 2010*, have not been evaluated by the United States Food and Drug Administration and are not approved to diagnose, treat, cure or prevent disease.

The information provided in the book, *How to Get Off Psychiatric Drugs Safely 2010*, is for informational purposes only and is not intended as a substitute for advice from your physician or other healthcare professional.

You should not use the information in this book for diagnosis or treatment of any health problem or for prescription of any medication or other treatment.

You should consult with a healthcare professional before starting any diet, exercise or supplementation program, before taking any medication, or if you have, or suspect that you might have a health problem.

James Harper is the Founder and President of The Road Back Program, a non-profit 501(c)3 Public Charity. Donations to The Road Back Program are tax deductable in the United States and Canada.

A NOTE FROM THE FOUNDER

Since 1999 when The Road Back Program, *How to Get Off Psychiatric Drugs Safely*, was released to the general public, tens of thousands of people have successfully tapered off their psychiatric medications using The Road Back Program.

I want to acknowledge the many people, from the four corners of Earth and all walks of life, who have successfully come off psychiatric medications using this program. Their perseverance and feedback have helped advance this program to today's high degree of success.

And I applaud you, opening this book for the first time, for your courage and resolve to change your life and get yourself back as your reward.

I understand the apprehension you may feel about deciding to come off psychiatric medications, especially if you have tried to do so before and failed, or if you have heard horror stories of others who have tried to come off their medications.

Further, I understand the questions you might be asking at this point:

- *Will I experience mental or physical pain while on this program?*

- *Will I have other side effects while on this program?*

- *Will the medication side effects get worse before they get better?*

- *Will my depression get worse during this program?*

- *Will my anxiety levels increase?*

You may have many other questions in addition to those above, but most importantly you should know that I have formulated The Road Back Program to be virtually side effect free. The testament to this, as you will see throughout the book, is that people just like you start to feel better, both mentally and physically, from day one.

The Road Back Program is simple, effective, and extremely powerful: when applied correctly. You too can have resounding success in getting off your psychiatric medications and getting your life back.

Based on extensive research, specific supplements have been formulated for this program. Their use, in conjunction with the full and complete Road Back Program, have resulted in an estimated 80% success rate of people getting off their psychiatric medications, while also enormously reducing the potential and feared side effects from withdrawal.

What unwanted feelings come from you and what feelings do the drugs generate? The Road Back Program separates these confusing symptoms, and once this separation occurs, the real you emerges.

One major change most people experience with The Road Back; their reach for life returns or truly begins for the first time. Reach is defined as: to extend out; to touch or to seize; to communicate with.

Life is defined as: the quality that distinguishes a *vital* and functional being from a dead body or inanimate matter (Webster's Dictionary). Per the definition of life, *you* are vital. We need you and humankind needs you. The positive changes you can bring to others are beyond imagining. Life can be grand, life can be fulfilling; you, changing your life and having "reach" return will absolutely affect others in your environment.

Reach can return with your children, spouse, work or activities you have been putting off for years that you have always wanted to do, or to do once again.

Remember and hold the following close to your heart as you travel The Road Back:

- You Can Change.

- You Can Change How You Feel.

- You Can Be a Positive Influence for Others.

- You Can Make It.

As you read this book, perhaps you might be thinking "...this sounds good for others..." or "...others can make it, but not me..." Believe me, I am referring directly to you.

My best to you in your journey,

Jim Harper
Founder
The Road Back

CONTENTS

1. The Road Back Basics 1

2. The Four Simple Steps 7

3. "Nutritionals" Used on The Road Back Program 11

4. Medication Side Effects 25

5. Things to Be Aware of... 59

6. General Pre-Tapering and Tapering Instructions............ 63

7. Daily Journal 77

8. Graph Your Success.. 81

9. Pre-Taper for Benzodiazepines, Anti-anxiety, Anticonvulsants and Sleep Medication......................... 83

10. Pre-Taper for Antidepressants, Antipsychotics, and ADHD Medications... 89

11. How to Taper Off Benzodiazepines, Anti-anxiety, Anticonvulsants and Sleep Medications 99

12. How to Taper Off Antidepressants, Antipychotics and ADHD Medication.. 103

13. Once Off Medication 109

14. What to Do if You Have Already Started to Taper Off Your Medication or Quit Cold Turkey.........................113

15. How to Taper Off Multiple Medications 117

16. What Can be Done if You Have Never Taken Psychiatric Medication... 123

17. The Science Behind The Road Back............................ 129

Glossary.. 147

References 183

CHAPTER 1

THE ROAD BACK BASICS

"When I first read your website, I thought no way. This is too simple. Barley? Give me a break. I figured I really didn't have anything to lose. I felt like crap warmed over anyway. Two weeks later and I mean two weeks later, I am a new man! The fog has cleared, the depression is gone, and my wife has a husband again. Barley, who would have thought? Needless to say, I was not surprised when the Omega 3 and Body Calm did exactly what you said they would. Thank you from the bottom of my big Texas heart."

T.D.

Austin, TX.

People from all over the world send in testimonials like this every day, praising The Road Back Program and how it has helped them regain their hold on life. Often, as this man said, the program at first seems too simple. When something is simple, there could be a tendency to disbelieve results. Nevertheless, the Road Back Program IS simple, while also highly effective when followed using the correct supplements, and completing all steps.

The Road Back Program is a very specific, heavily researched, proven program. As noted above, I formulated this program to help people get off all kinds of drugs, while reducing to almost zero the crippling side effects often associated with coming off the drugs.

Newly formulated psychiatric medications seem to incessantly roll out of research labs into distribution. But I have found over the years that no matter what the drug's formulation, The Road Back Program is still effective. Since you are reading this book you most likely understand, firsthand, the devastating side effects of psychiatric medications. As of today, tens of thousands of people over the world have used The Road Back Program to free themselves from those crippling bonds.

Which Side Effects Are You Suffering From?

Due to the widely varying circumstances of the many people who will read this book, I have outlined several scenarios delineating where you might now stand, and how The Road Back Program will apply to you. Establishing your current particular circumstances will be of great benefit and provide a starting point for your progress on The Road Back Program.

Scenario One:
You are not on any psychiatric medications, and never have been, but are thinking about taking these medications:

Debate and statistics hit the news nearly every day about the effectiveness or potential harm caused by psychiatric drugs. The confusions tend to mount further when the latest clinical trial results counters the evidence published just last month.

I am not about to enter the fray of the psychiatric drug debate with this book. The intent here is to offer hope and solutions for those desiring to safely taper off psychiatric medication as well as offer a few solutions to those seeking an alternative to psychiatric medication.

If you are looking for a solution rather than taking a psychiatric drug, this book offers nutritional answers and a simple blood test that may provide the better way you are seeking. That word "may," should be capitalized, italicized, underlined, put in bold type and double-sized.

Certainly, while nutrition is not the answer for all of the ills that might beset our lives, neither is a drug the answer.

If your symptoms are caused or perpetuated by deficiencies in a specific or broad range of vitamins, amino acids, fatty acids, enzymes, protein, etc, then this part of the program will probably be the answer for you.

Scenario Two:
You are on one or more psychiatric medications and want to withdraw from these drugs:

You are a prime candidate for The Road Back Program. You may or may not be experiencing side effects from your medications. You may or may not have tried to taper before. You may have been on your medications for a few days or many years.

You will find tremendous benefit and success with The Road Back Program.

Scenario Three:
You have started to taper off and are suffering:

Dr. Donald E. McAlpine, Psychiatry and Psychology, Mayo Clinic notes: *"It's important to taper off slowly, extending the taper over several weeks under your physician's direction. When you stop too quickly, you may experience so-called discontinuation symptoms, which can masquerade as relapse."*

The Road Back Program has been designed to help you get back on track and succeed with the tapering process. This can take a little more time initially, but there IS a way back.

Scenario Four:
You have already tapered off your medications and are still suffering, or stopped the medication "cold turkey":

Due to the nature and composition of psychiatric medications and their effects on the body, withdrawal side effects can plague you long after complete withdrawal. Such "protracted" or continuing withdrawal side effects are probably the most difficult situation to deal with. The Road Back Program can be effective and successful in eliminating these side effects from your life.

Stopping your medication "cold turkey" or tapering off too quickly cause many of the same side effects, and often to the same magnitude. This situation usually requires the longest road back, but can be accomplished. Many people start to feel better one week into the program and reach a major positive change by the fourteenth day of the program.

Scenario Five:
You have all four of the points listed below:

In the past, The Road Back could not help a person who fit the following four points. Today we have a program for you as well.

These four points are:

1. You are sensitive to all supplements and most foods.

2. You came off your medications and suffered *extreme* withdrawal symptoms.

3. You are still experiencing "protracted" withdrawals, even though off your medications.

4. You have been off your medications for at least six months.

There was a time The Road Back Program would not help a person within Scenario Five. Research breakthroughs during 2010 now allows a person that falls in this category to have a very good chance of recovery.

I urge you to not give up hope. This program should get you fully recovered from the medication.

CHAPTER 2

THE FOUR SIMPLE STEPS

"My God! I took the Power Barley and the Omega 3 this morning and it is as if thousands of pounds of weight were just lifted from my body. I feel bright, energetic but not hyper. This is truly amazing. I read the testimonials on your website, and thought maybe for other people this works, but I have tried supplements before. Your wording of well-being now makes sense. I can say for the first time ever I know what it feels like to have the feeling of well-being. It is Christmas morning where I am and I can't thank you enough for the unexpected present."

P.M.
Medford, OR.

Step One

Do Not Stop Your Medications Abruptly
- Do not "self medicate" (adjust the medication dosage without consulting your prescribing physician).

- Do not think you are somehow "different" regarding your medications and think you can cut your medications by 50%, drop two meds at one time or skip days of the medication, etc.
- Keep it simple; follow the program.
- If you are doing well and seeing results, do not change anything. Just stay on the program.
- Remember that The Road Back Program is a systematic process.

Step Two

Find Out What You Will Need for the Program

- Read Chapters 3 through 8.

- If you are taking a benzodiazepine, sleep, anticonvulsant or pain medications read and follow Chapter 9.

- If you are taking an antidepressant, antipsychotic or ADHD medication read and follow Chapter 10.

- If you are on a medication from both the above categories read and follow Chapter 10.

- If you have already started to taper or quit your medication cold turkey read and follow Chapter 14.

Step Three

Get a Complete Physical

- Schedule a complete physical with your doctor.

- Take this book with you and review the program with your doctor.

- Have your physician rule out any physical illness or disease.

Step Four

Purchase Your Supplements and Get Started

- Call TRB Health offices 1 + (866) 810-3809, or go to *www.trbhealth.com*, and purchase the supplements needed for your personal program.

- We offer free support with this program. Please do not hesitate to call us or send an e-mail with questions. We will not give medical advice; however, we will guide you through the steps and stay with you throughout. You can call us at 1 + (866) 892-0238.

CHAPTER 3

"NUTRITIONALS" USED
ON THE ROAD BACK PROGRAM

"I am now more than halfway off my antidepressant, using the program. I was able to reduce a little bit of the medication with my naturopath, but we reached a standstill after the second reduction. The side effects started and we could not get rid of them. The Omega 3 got rid of the brain zaps within a few hours and they never came back. The Body Calm has been amazing at helping me stay calm during the day and with my sleep. And that barley did just what you said it would do for my energy and complete feelings. I can't thank you enough."

J.S.
New York

The Basic Nutritional Premise

The body is an amazing and complex instrument, designed to deal with the rigors of life, as long as it is cared for properly. However, when the body's chemistry or systems are altered, the body will fight back to balance out the attack.

Bringing back that balance is critical if a person is taking a psychoactive medication.

Over the past decade, I have spent thousands of hours researching the correct and most basic nutrient system for this program. The year 2010, has brought the next generation of research to application. The 2010 edition of this book makes the program even more effective, easier to follow and reduces the time it takes to get off psychoactive medication.

A few examples of clinical trials: antidepressants cause insulin resistance and prolonged use of benzodiazepines depletes the body of the B vitamin biotin. These two examples give an indication of how one might treat medication side effects and why a few supplements are part of this program.

In other words, if you have taken a benzodiazepine for an extended period of time and you have depression and/or tingling or numbness of the extremities, you are very well deficient in biotin and adding biotin to your daily routine will handle the symptom if the deficiency is the cause.

The list of symptoms associated with insulin resistance is quite long. Diabetes and obesity are two of the final results of being insulin resistant but there are other symptoms a person will begin experiencing before the onset of the conditions.

When a person puts back the correct nutrients in the body and allows the body to begin balancing itself once again the positive changes a person feels can be vast and dramatic.

How The Program Works

Your body naturally triggers a self-protective inflammatory process. This natural function responds to normal activities such as exercise, fighting off toxins, allergies, illness, incorrect foods, weight gain, medications - you name it.

For example, a sore throat or infected cut. The area becomes red and inflamed as the body rushes microscopic "fire fighters" to the area to contain and put out the fire and to then start the healing process.

But if your body gets overloaded and can no longer control the inflammation, or lacks enough "fire fighters" to douse the flames, then an internal switch flips, and your systems can start going awry, ultimately resulting in an overall imbalance.

If you have a physical condition, including menopause, weight gain, diabetes or so many others, and then throw most psychoactive medications on top, you can be adding fuel to an already burning fire. In essence, you flip the switch that overloads your body so it can no longer function as intended.

However, and a big however; using supplements, specifically antioxidants incorrectly, in the wrong amount, combination, or the time of day taken, can cause more harm than help.

The body will produce and release substances called cytokines when the immune system is activated. Depending on your body, these cytokines may have been overly active before you started taking medication or they may have been inhibited once the medication was started. We all react differently when medication is taken. One thing is common though with all of us, that is the need to maintain or to get back to a natural body balance.

Oxidative stress will be significantly higher in the body of anyone diagnosed with anxiety, depression, bipolar, schizophrenia, ADHD and OCD. The brain is most susceptible to oxidative stress and a multitude of clinical trials have shown significantly higher oxidative stress in the brain of bipolar and schizophrenic patients. The supplement called JNK will help stop the oxidative stress before it even starts.

The area of nutrition is littered with confusing words and information so technical, it can seem overwhelming. I have tried to simplify and distill what you need to know, so you can proceed with the program while understanding the basic premise and how your body works to counteract the imbalances created by the medication.

Thousands of people worldwide have stood where you now stand; ready to take their lives back and free themselves from psychoactive medication and the resulting side effects. While every person is unique and life offers no guarantees, if you follow this program precisely, you should begin to feel better and do better soon after you start.

> *"I started your program two weeks ago and what a differ-ence! I didn't think you were telling the truth about the prod-ucts, but I feel like a new woman. Can I stay on the products for life after the taper is over? Thank you for your efforts. You all are a godsend"*
>
> *L.V.*
>
> *Reno, Nevada*

When I started my research into the psychoactive drug-tapering problem, I relied on available, over-the-counter nutritional products to help people with their tapering. As with any other research, there were ups and downs to this approach, because over-the-counter nutritional products were often either too harsh, or just not of the quality needed to accomplish the task. However, there were a few supplements found that were fully backed by clinical science and each bottle label matched exactly what was inside of the bottle.

What I found is that throwing random, unrelated health products into your body during any form of withdrawal from psychoactive medication, would create at best, a "willy-nilly," disordered, unpre-dictable response, or in the worst case scenario extreme illness. While some *might* benefit from such an approach, the vast majority will not achieve the desired results, even worse, they could create new problems for themselves in the process.

My goal is to help you safely taper off psychoactive medication, while dramatically reducing the side effects of your medication, as well as the side effects of withdrawal.

What works are the correct "nutrients" introduced into your body in the correct amounts at the correct times throughout the day, so the side effects of the medication and the tapering process are minimized, while concurrently the relief is increased.

Specific "nutrients," taken in an exact order at specific times will counter-balance and eliminate the side effects.

Supplements Used in the Program

Body Calm

One of the most common complaints of people on either psychoactive medication or those who are trying to come off their medication is daytime anxiety and the inability to achieve a normal sleep at night. Sleep is an integral part of life, it helps to stabilize mood, foster clear thinking and assist with reaction time. Sleep gives the body a chance to rebuild. Even though your body is doing a lot of work while you sleep, you should not be. Without plenty of restful sleep, daily functioning can be miserable.

Different from any prescribed medication you may be on or have taken in the past, Body Calm does not knock you out or turn you into a zombie. Taken during the day, Body Calm will help relieve anxiety without making you tired, foggy or having a feeling of not being there. Body Calm taken at night, about an hour before bed, will help you fall asleep naturally. Upon waking in the morning, you should not feel groggy, weary or have to drag yourself out of the sheets.

The ingredient in Body Calm is a tart cherry, made into a powdered form and put in a veggie capsule. This type of tart cherry is a COX-2 enzyme inhibitor. Stress during our daily life promotes the production of the enzyme COX-2 and inhibiting this enzyme reduces the anxiety associated with stress.

Body Calm Supreme

Severe anxiety, stress and insomnia are common withdrawal side effects, comprising the most common side effects for all psychoactive medication, especially during withdrawal. Body Calm Supreme was formulated for use in conjunction with Body Calm to handle anxiety, stress and insomnia. Body Calm Supreme combines 50 mg Body Calm and 200 mg of the herb passion flower.

You might be tempted to go to your local store or search online and purchase a passion flower supplement. It is strongly suggested that you only use the TRB Health brand of passion flower. There are over 500 species of passion flower and Body Calm Supreme is only made from one of the species. The herb extraction process is completely different from other passion flower supplements and the strength of Body Calm Supreme is the highest you can find. This is why only 200 mg of passion flower is needed in a capsule.

Passion Flower has been shown in several clinical trials during the past decades to handle such things as generalized anxiety, insomnia, hypertension, withdrawal off benzodiazepines, withdrawal off opiates, narcotics, alcohol and several other addictive substances. Every clinical trial was successful. The same type of passion flower used in the clinical trials has been used to formulate Body Calm Supreme.

JNK

The JNK supplement is a combination of nutritional supplements in veggie capsules in a packet. There are 30-packets in each bottle and you will take 1 packet first thing in the morning.

The human body has a gene called JNK and the supplement is named after the gene. When the JNK gene becomes over activated a person will likely feel additional stress, anxiety or panic attacks, gain weight, feel depressed or any of the hundreds of medication side effects.

Antidepressants actually make the JNK gene more active and this activation has been found to be the cause of antidepressant induced diabetes or insulin resistance at the very least.

People diagnosed with mood disorders are usually prescribed Lithium, Depakote or any of the common drugs prescribed for this feeling. The drugs are actively suppressing the over activation of the JNK gene. When these drugs work for a person, the suppression of the JNK gene is why they work.

If you have gained weight while taking medications, the answer and solution will be the JNK supplement and the JNK Liquid Booster. Just take 1 packet of the JNK supplement in the morning along with the JNK Liquid Booster a few hours later and experience weight loss for what might be the first time in years.

The JNK supplement is used in all taper programs and if you are not taking a psychoactive medication the JNK supplement is the most vital supplement of all to take. The list of symptoms and body conditions that will no longer exist when the JNK gene is inhibited would require a separate book to list them all.

Power Barley Formula

The Power Barley Formula is comprised of three simple yet powerful ingredients: young green barley, Aktivated Barley™, and carrots all blended into an easily assimilated powdered form. Easy assimilation is key to the nutritional effectiveness of this product.

Power Barley Formula is U.S.D.A. approved and certified 100% organic. Based on the contents of this formula and an FDA issued statement in December 2005, TRB Health can make the following health claim regarding the Power Barley Formula: "Soluble fiber from foods, such as Power Barley Formula, as part of a diet low in saturated fat and cholesterol, may reduce the risk of heart disease. A serving of Power Barley Formula supplies two grams of the soluble fiber necessary per day to have this effect."

Power Barley Formula is only used if you are taking an antidepressant, have fatigue and do not have daytime anxiety or insomnia.

Omega 3 Supreme

The use of omega 3 fish oil is now scientifically documented, through a multitude of clinical trials to help people overcome the symptoms associated with several psychiatric disorders. The successful trials have used an omega 3 fish oil that is higher in EPA than DHA content. The EPA fraction of the fish oil helps with brain function. When a person is taking a psychoactive drug, specifically antidepressants, ADHD medication and antipsychotics, the uptake and turnover of the fatty acids can be altered and that results in head side effects.

EPA enhances the electrical functions and communication between all the systems in your brain, which your body relies on to function properly.

DHA helps build the brain structurally, and as such, is a much-needed nutrient for the correct brain formation during growth. Both EPA and DHA are critical compounds for a person on psychoactive medications. With these compounds stripped from the body, the communications or electrical impulses from one nerve ending to another do not flow smoothly, but rather jump in all directions creating such things as "brain zaps," "fogginess," irritability, agitation, forgetfulness and more.

The amount of EPA and DHA taken during your taper will directly affect how well, or how poorly, you do on the program.

If you will be tapering off an anti-depressant, anti-psychotic, or ADHD medication, it is doubly important that you use the correct quantity and quality of omega 3 fish oil. The Omega 3 Supreme fish oil sold by TRB Health was specifically created for high EPA and has been cleaned of toxins generally associated with fish oil.

Beyond the benefits listed above, omega 3 fish oil will also help stop the over activation of the JNK gene!

Vitamin E

Vitamin E is commonly found in regular foods, such as vegetable oils, nuts, whole grains and leafy vegetables. As discussed earlier, though found in many foods consumed on a regular basis it is difficult, if not impossible, to derive the total Vitamin E needed from diet alone.

Further, pollution, fried foods, bad carbohydrates, drugs, birth control pills, hormone replacement therapy and so many other bad influences test the vitamin E that we do have in our bodies. Vitamin E is an anti-oxidant, a natural compound that protects the body from toxins, and also helps protect other anti-oxidants in the body from being destroyed. It further helps the body eliminate circulating toxins or poisons. When taking the Power Barley Formula you are causing a mild detoxification process – a good thing. Vitamin E helps your body neutralize these toxins and as these toxins are removed from the body you will start to feel better with more energy.

The components making a complete vitamin and distinguishing available vitamin E's are staggering, having filled volumes. This program assists a person off medication and in the process ensures there will be no drug/supplement interactions with our recommendations. Beyond the correct mixture of vitamin E is the quality or purity of a natural vitamin E. Some forms of vitamin E will create higher plasma concentrations of vitamin E while other forms will create vitamin E in the tissue. While Vitamin E is an antioxidant, the incorrect vitamin E can become an oxidant and cause inflammation and in some cases create a drug/supplement interaction.

The A.C. Grace Company has been manufacturing vitamin E for more than 46 years. We recommend their Unique E with mixed tocopherols because of their manufacturing process.

Optional Supplements

There are optional supplements that can be used to help with specific symptoms. I have found 80% of the people we work with on the program do just fine with the supplements listed earlier, but 20% needed a little extra help with specific symptoms. I have listed the optional supplements below and what they can be used for.

Beta 1, 3-D Glucan

The human immune system includes a substance called IL-2. Individuals with low levels of IL-2 will have anxiety and problems with sleep. Stage 2 of sleep requires a sufficient level of IL-2 for a deep restful sleep.

Beta 1, 3-D Glucan has been clinically proven to not only increase levels of IL-2 in the human immune system but also to keep the IL-2 levels increased for an extended time after the product is discontinued.

If you have anxiety and or insomnia, use the Body Calm and Body Calm Supreme first and if these symptoms do not subside within 2 weeks you may have low IL-2 and supplementing with the Beta 1, 3-D Glucan would be in order. Taking three of the 100 mg capsules in the morning will usually do the trick.

Biotin

The B vitamin biotin is used in the program if you have taken a benzodiazepine or any anti-anxiety medication for an extended period. What an extended period is, is a subjective time in the clinical trials, so you will need to determine the need of biotin based on your symptoms. If you are taking a benzodiazepine or anti-anxiety medication and have depression and or a tingling or numbness of the extremities, the odds are very high you have been depleted of biotin by the medication and you should include biotin during the program. The biotin from TRB Health is a pure grade biotin and the capsules are a therapeutic strength at 5,000 mcg a capsule. Taking 1 capsule in the morning may be all you need. Results happen within 3 days if you are taking the correct amount of biotin. Some people may need 3 capsules a day, morning, noon and again around 5 pm.

B6, B12 and Folate

B6, B12 and folate will be deficient in most diets of the 21st century. The ramifications of this deficiency may be one of the factors associated with the high percentage of the population experiencing prolonged depression. Several clinical trials have shown low levels of these 3 required vitamins to be directly related to depression and the severity of the depression.

Clinical trials have also shown antidepressants to be more effective when the patient also takes B6, B12 and folate along with the antidepressant. We will let others debate if the successful result is only from the B6, B12 and folate or if the success really comes from the combination of supplement and medication.

The master antioxidant glutathione plays a critical role with detoxification of all toxins. There are several ways to increase glutathione levels in the body but the most natural way is to have ample B6, B12 and folate levels and the body will convert certain amino acids to help production of glutathione.

CalesiumD

CalesiumD is a proprietary blend of calcium citrate, magnesium and a trace of vitamin D3. The calcium's non-ionic form reduces the chance of calcium induced anxiety or insomnia. Many people taking medication are calcium deficient and have a need for calcium but an ionic form of calcium causes increased anxiety. For the best absorption of calcium, include a pre-biotic called Calsorption.

Essential Protein Formula

The Essential Protein Formula is excellent when you have anxiety or insomnia. This product is also effective when you are having a problem with blood sugar and that is part of the anxiety or insomnia problem.

TRB Health misnamed their Essential Protein Formula completely. Please do not believe you should go to a store and purchase a whey protein for this program. The whey protein in this formula is no more than a base for other nutritionals to be added for easy mixing. The real benefit of the formula comes from a type of barley in the product, as well as wheat germ and lecithin.

Probiotic Supreme

Clinical trials have shown that at least 18% of the people who have taken an antidepressant have Candida yeast overgrowth. Three possible side effects of Candida yeast overgrowth are *depression, weight gain and bloating*. If you have ever used an antibiotic, a birth control pill, or most other medications, you have immensely increased the chance of Candida yeast overgrowth.

Other symptoms of Candida yeast overgrowth include – fatigue, recurring infections, mental fog, headaches, sore throat, abdominal pain, muscle tension and pain, joint pain or swelling, as well as digestive issues, such as heartburn, indigestion and Irritable Bowel Syndrome (IBS).

RenewPro

To further lower the inflammation marker IL-6, remove toxins and supply the body with all natural amino acids, you can use a product called RenewPro. A complete book could be written on RenewPro and what it does within the human body.

First, RenewPro contains an exceptional amount of the amino acid cysteine. Cysteine lowers IL-6 significantly. RenewPro will greatly increase the intracellular levels of our master antioxidant glutathione. Glutathione will also help lower IL-6. A protein called lactoferrin is higher in RenewPro than any other whey protein product. Lactoferrin lowers IL-6.

If you are lacking energy or feeling dull, RenewPro is worth the try.

RenewPro is a whey protein concentrate made from disease-free, pesticide-free, chemical-free, hormone treatment-free and natural grass pasture fed cows.

Packages and individual supplements are available at TRB Health. www.trbhealth.com or 1-866-810-3809.

I do not sell the supplements and neither does The Road Back Program. The supplements are made by a high quality vitamin manufacturer, TRB Health, located in Florida, U.S.A.

CHAPTER 4

MEDICATION SIDE EFFECTS

Side Effects of Psychiatric Medications

The psychiatric medications we are dealing with are classified as psychotropic – having ability or quality of altering emotions, perceptions, behaviors, and bodily functions – especially true of certain drugs.

This chapter lists many possible side effects experienced from either taking these drugs, or when trying to withdraw from them. If you, or anyone you know, are taking any of these medications the "real you" could well be buried under some of the following symptoms. But rest assured, no one has all of these side effects, and no single drug or combination of these drugs can produce all the side effects listed here.

You may know from experience that a single withdrawal side effect can be horrifying. And if you, or anyone you know, have ever had a bad withdrawal experience you would probably rather sign up for open-heart surgery without anesthesia than suffer those side effects again. And for this very reason, many people who have contacted The Road Back are gun shy at the very thought of withdrawing from medication. Before The Road Back Program you were faced with a quandary: suffer the side effects of the drugs, or gut it out and suffer the side effects of withdrawal.

The Road Back Program eliminates these worries and concerns by reducing to almost zero the side effects of withdrawal, so that you can come off your medication(s) smoothly and easily.

The following list is broken down into categories, covering the various areas of the body, such as the nervous system, lymph system, emotional and mental symptoms and so forth. These categories will make it easier for you to find the part of the body or system that you are interested in, or want to know more about.

In this list you will find many physical ailments and complaints, as well as emotional or mental symptoms that people experience every day because of a specific medical condition. These symptoms and ailments may be the reason that you started psychiatric medications, or conversely, these medications may actually be causing the negative symptoms you are experiencing now.

This unknown catches almost everyone, doctor and patient alike, off guard. So the question that needs to be answered in order for you to proceed with The Road Back Program is: Are you dealing with a physical condition that needs to be treated medically or with a by-product symptom of the psychiatric medication(s) you are taking?

Getting Your Doctor's Approval

Because of the overload and damage potentially caused by psychiatric medications, your body in general, and your immune system in particular, are in a weakened condition, and can thus leave you open to infections and disease. On the other hand, you may be taking prescription medications for actual physical conditions, which could be contra-indicated in terms of doing The Road Back Program. These could include blood thinners and heart medication, as well as clotting agents.

Products used in The Road Back Program include Omega 3 and vitamin E, which could both be contra-indicated if taking heart medications or blood thinners. Additionally, some of the products contain naturally occurring, (not synthetic) vitamin K, which could be contra-indicated if taking any type of blood clotting medication.

For these reasons, consult your doctor *before* starting any part of this program to sort out, or discover and correctly determine, whether you are a candidate for The Road Back Program.

After you have ruled out any *real* medical problem, you will know that if any strange symptom begins during The Road Back Program, you are most likely experiencing something caused by the psychiatric medications you are taking. Such will be true for both emotional and physical symptoms.

The following list does not include all possible side effects from psychoactive medication. Using the Freedom of Information Act, I received all side effects associated with a popular antidepressant medication during clinical trials. The list is long enough to make this book be double the size if they were included. The side effects in this chapter are the most common.

The first list of side effects in this chapter are for antidepressants, antipsychotics and ADHD medications. On page 46 of this chapter you will find benzodiazepine, anti-anxiety and sleep medication side effects.

SIDE EFFECTS OF ANTIDEPRESSANTS, ANTIPSYCHOTICS AND ADHD MEDICATION

GENERAL BODY

Dry Mouth - Less moisture in the mouth than is usual.

Increased Sweating - A large quantity of perspiration that is medically caused.

Allergy - Extreme sensitivity of body tissues triggered by substances in the air, drugs, or foods causing a variety of reactions such as sneezing, itching, asthma, hay fever, skin rashes, nausea and/or vomiting.

Asthenia - A physically weak condition.

Chest Pains - Severe discomfort in the chest caused by not enough oxygen going to the heart because of blood vessel narrowing or spasms.

Chills - Appearing pale while cold and shivering. Sometimes accompanied by fever.

Edema of Extremities - Abnormal swelling of body tissue caused by the collection of fluid.

Fall - Suddenly losing a normal standing upright position.

Fatigue - Loss of normal strength thus not able to do usual physical and mental activities.

Fever - Abnormally high body temperature, normal being 98.6 degrees Fahrenheit or 37 degrees Centigrade. Fever is a symptom of disease or disorder in the body. The body is affected by feeling hot, chilled, sweaty, weak and exhausted. If the fever goes too high or lasts too long, death can result.

Hot Flashes - Brief, abnormal enlargement of the blood vessels that causes a sudden heat sensation over the entire body. Sometimes experienced by menopausal women.

Influenza (Flu)-like Symptoms - Demonstrating irritation of the respiratory tract (organs of breathing) such as a cold, sudden fever, aches and pains, as well as feeling weak and seeking bed rest, which is similar to having the flu.

Leg Pain - A hurtful sensation in the legs caused by excessive stimulation of the nerve endings in the legs, resulting in extreme discomfort.

Malaise - The somewhat unclear feeling of discomfort when a person starts to feel sick.

Pain in Limb - Sudden, sharp and uncontrolled leg or arm discomfort.

Syncope - A short period of light-headedness or unconsciousness (black-out) also known as fainting, caused by lack of oxygen to the brain because of an interruption in blood flow to the brain.

Tightness of Chest - Mild or sharp discomfort, tightness or pressure in the chest area (anywhere between the throat and belly). The causes can be mild or seriously life-threatening because they include the heart, lungs and surrounding muscles.

CARDIOVASCULAR
(INVOLVING THE HEART AND THE BLOOD VESSELS)

Palpitation - Unusual and abnormal heartbeat that is sometimes irregular, but rapid, and forceful thumping or fluttering. It can be brought on by shock, excitement, exertion or medical stimulants. A person is normally unaware of his/her heartbeat.

Hypertension - High blood pressure, a symptom of disease in the blood vessels leading away from the heart. Hypertension is known as the "silent killer." The symptoms are usually not obvious; however, it can lead to damage to the heart, brain, kidneys and eyes, and can even lead to stroke and kidney failure.

Bradycardia - The heart rate is slowed from around 72 beats per minute, which is normal, to below 60 beats per minute in an adult.

Tachycardia - The heart rate speeds up to above 100 beats per minute in an adult. Normal adult heart rate average is 72 beats per minute.

ECG Abnormal - A test called an electrocardiogram (ECG) records the activity of the heart by measuring heartbeats as well as the position and size of the heart's four chambers. An ECG also measures whether there is damage to the heart and the effects of drugs or mechanical devices like a heart pacemaker. When the test is abnormal this means one or more of the following are present: heart disease, defects, beating too fast or too slow, disease of the blood vessels leading from the heart or the heart valves, and/or a past or impending heart attack.

Flushing - Skin all over the body turns red.

Varicose Veins - Unusually swollen veins near the surface of the skin that sometimes appear twisted and knotted, but always enlarged. They are called hemorrhoids when appearing around the rectum. The cause is attributed to hereditary weakness in the veins aggravated by obesity, pregnancy, pressure from standing, aging, etc. Severe cases may develop swelling in the legs, ankles and feet, eczema and/or ulcers in the affected areas.

GASTROINTESTINAL
(INVOLVING THE STOMACH AND THE INTESTINES)

Abdominal Cramp/Pain - Sudden, severe, uncontrollable and painful shortening and thickening of the muscles in the belly. The belly includes the stomach, as well as the intestines, liver, kidneys, pancreas, spleen, gall bladder and urinary bladder.

Belching - Noisy release of gas from the stomach through the mouth; a burp.

Bloating - Swelling of the belly caused by excessive intestinal gas.

Constipation - Difficulty in having a bowel movement where the material in the bowels is hard due to a lack of exercise, fluid intake, or roughage in the diet or due to certain drugs.

Diarrhea - Unusually frequent and excessive runny bowel movements that may result in severe dehydration and shock.

Dyspepsia/Indigestion - The discomfort one may experience after eating. Can be heartburn, gas, nausea, a bellyache or bloating.

Flatulence - More gas than normal in the digestive organs.

Gagging - Involuntary choking and/or involuntary vomiting.

Gastritis - A severe irritation of the mucus lining of the stomach, either short in duration or lasting for a long period of time.

Gastroenteritis - A condition in which the membranes of the stomach and intestines are irritated.

Gastrointestinal Hemorrhage - Excessive internal bleeding in the stomach and intestines.

Gastro Esophageal Reflux - A continuous state where stomach juices flow back into the throat causing acid indigestion and heartburn and possibly injury to the throat.

Heartburn - A burning pain in the area of the breastbone caused by stomach juices flowing back up into the throat.

Hemorrhoids - Small rounded purplish swollen veins that bleed, itch or are painful and appear around the anus.

Increased Stool Frequency - see "Diarrhea."

Indigestion - Inability to properly consume and absorb food in the digestive tract, causing constipation, nausea, stomachache, gas, swollen belly, pain and general discomfort or sickness.

Nausea - Stomach irritation with a queasy sensation similar to motion sickness and a feeling that one is going to vomit.

Polyposis Gastric - Tumors that grow on stems in the lining of the stomach, which usually become cancerous.

Swallowing Difficulty - A feeling that food is stuck in the throat or upper chest area and won't go down, making it difficult to swallow.

Toothache - Pain in a tooth above and below the gum line.

Vomiting - Involuntarily throwing up the contents of the stomach, usually accompanied by a nauseated, sick feeling just prior to doing so.

HEMIC & LYMPHATIC
(INVOLVING THE BLOOD AND THE CLEAR FLUIDS
IN THE TISSUES THAT CONTAIN WHITE BLOOD CELLS)

Anemia - A condition in which the blood is no longer carrying enough oxygen, so the person looks pale and easily gets dizzy, weak and tired. More severely, a person can end up with an abnormal heart, as well as breathing and digestive difficulties.

Bruise - Damage to the skin resulting in a purple-green-yellow skin coloration that is caused by breaking of the blood vessels in the area without breaking the surface of the skin.

Nosebleed - Blood loss from the nose.

Hematoma - Broken blood vessels that cause a swelling in an area on the body.

Lymphadenopathy Cervical - The lymph nodes in the neck, part of the body's immune system, become swollen and enlarged by reacting to the presence of a drug. The swelling is the result of the white blood cells multiplying in order to fight the invasion of the drug.

METABOLIC & NUTRITIONAL (ENERGY AND HEALTH)

Arthralgia - Sudden sharp nerve pain in one or more joints.

Arthropathy - Joint disease or abnormal joints.

Arthritis - Painfully inflamed and swollen joints. The reddened and swollen condition is brought on by a serious injury or shock to the body either from physical or emotional causes.

Back Discomfort - Severe physical distress in the area from the neck to the pelvis along the backbone.

Bilirubin Increased - Bilirubin is a waste product of the break-down of old blood cells. Bilirubin is sent to the liver to be made water-soluble so it can be eliminated from the body through empty-ing the bladder. A drug can interfere with or damage this normal liver function, creating liver disease.

Decreased Weight - Uncontrolled and measured loss of heaviness or weight.

Gout - A severe arthritis condition that is caused by the dumping of a waste product called uric acid into the tissues and joints. It can worsen and cause the body to develop a deformity after going through stages of pain, inflammation, severe tenderness and stiffness.

Hepatic Enzymes Increased - An increase in the amount of paired liver proteins that regulate liver processes causing a condition in which the liver functions abnormally.

Hypercholesterolemia - Too much cholesterol in the blood cells.

Hyperglycemia - An unhealthy amount of sugar in the blood.

Increased Weight - A concentration and storage of fat in the body accumulating over a period of time caused by unhealthy eating patterns, a lack of physical activity, or an inability to process food correctly, which can predispose the body to many disorders and diseases.

Jaw Pain - Pain due to irritation and swelling of the nerves associated with the mouth area where it opens and closes just in front of the ear. Some of the symptoms are: pain when chewing, headaches, loss of balance, stuffy ears or ringing in the ears and teeth grinding.

Jaw Stiffness - The result of squeezing and grinding the teeth while asleep that can cause teeth to deteriorate, as well as the muscles and joints of the jaw.

Joint Stiffness - A loss of free motion and easy flexibility where any two bones come together.

Muscle Cramp - When muscles contract uncontrollably without warning and do not relax. The muscles of any body organs can cramp.

Muscle Stiffness - The tightening of muscles making it difficult to bend.

Muscle Weakness - Loss of physical strength.

Myalgia - A general widespread pain and tenderness of the muscles.

Thirst - A strong, unnatural craving for moisture/water in the mouth and throat.

NERVOUS SYSTEM (SENSORY CHANNELS)

Carpal Tunnel Syndrome - A pinched nerve in the wrist that causes pain, tingling, and numbing.

Coordination Abnormal - A lack of normal, harmonious interaction of the parts of the body when it is in motion.

Dizziness - Losing one's balance while feeling unsteady and lightheaded. May lead to fainting.

Disequilibrium - Lack of mental and emotional balance.

Faintness - A temporary condition in which one is likely to become unconscious and fall.

Headache - A sharp or dull persistent pain in the head.

Hyperreflexia - A not normal (abnormal) and involuntary increased response in the tissues connecting the bones to the muscles.

Light-Headed Feeling - An uncontrolled and usually brief loss of consciousness usually caused by a lack of oxygen to the brain.

Migraine - Recurring severe head pain sometimes accompanied by nausea, vomiting, dizziness, flashes or spots before the eyes and ringing in the ears.

Muscle Contractions Involuntary - A spontaneous and uncontrollable tightening reaction of the muscles caused by electrical impulses from the nervous system.

Muscular Tone Increased - Uncontrolled and exaggerated muscle tension. Muscles are normally partially tensed which is what gives muscle tone.

Paresthesia - Burning, prickly, itchy, or tingling skin with no obvious or understood physical cause.

Restless Legs - A need to move the legs without any apparent reason. Sometimes there is pain, twitching, jerking, cramping, burning or a creepy-crawly sensation associated with the movements. It worsens when a person is inactive, and can interrupt sleep so one feels the need to move to gain some relief.

Shaking - Uncontrolled quivering and trembling as if one is cold and chilled.

Sluggishness - Lack of alertness and energy, as well as being slow to respond or perform in life.

Tics - A contraction of a muscle causing a repeated movement not under the control of the person, usually on the face or limbs.

Tremor - A nervous and involuntary vibrating or quivering of the body.

Twitching - Sharp, jerky and spastic motion, sometimes with a sharp sudden pain.

Vertigo - A sensation of dizziness with disorientation and confusion.

MENTAL AND EMOTIONAL

Aggravated Nervousness - A progressively worsening, irritated, and troubled state of mind.

Agitation - A suddenly violent and forceful emotionally disturbed state of mind.

Amnesia - Long or short term, partial or full memory loss created by emotional or physical shock, severe illness, or a blow to the head where the person was caused pain and became unconscious.

Anxiety Attack - Sudden and intense feelings of fear, terror, and dread, physically creating shortness of breath, sweating, trembling and heart palpitations.

Apathy - Complete lack of concern or interest for things that ordinarily would be regarded as important or would normally cause concern.

Appetite Decreased - Lack of appetite despite the ordinary caloric demands of living, with a resulting unintentional loss of weight.

Appetite Increased - An unusual hunger causing one to overeat.

Auditory Hallucination - Hearing things without the voices or noises being present.

Bruxism - Grinding and clenching of teeth while sleeping.

Carbohydrate Craving - A drive or craving to eat foods rich in sugar and starches (sweets, snacks and junk foods) that intensifies as the diet becomes more and more unbalanced due to the unbalancing of the proper nutritional requirements of the body.

Concentration Impaired - Unable to easily focus attention for long periods of time.

Confusion - Inability to think clearly or understand, preventing logical decision making.

Crying (Abnormal) - Unusual fits of weeping for short or long periods of time for no apparent reason.

Depersonalization - A condition in which one has lost a normal sense of personal identity.

Depression - A hopeless feeling of failure, loss and sadness that can deteriorate into thoughts of death. A very common reaction to or side effect of psychiatric drugs.

Disorientation - A loss of sense of direction, place, time or surroundings, as well as mental confusion regarding one's personal identity.

Dreaming (Abnormal) - Dreaming that leaves a very clear, detailed picture and impression when awake that can last for a long period of time and sometimes be unpleasant.

Emotional Lability - Suddenly breaking out in laughter or crying or doing both without being able to control the outburst of emotion. These episodes are unstable as they are caused by experiences or events that normally would not have this effect on an individual.

Excitability - Uncontrollably responding to stimuli (one's environment).

Feeling Unreal - The awareness that one has an undesirable emotion like fear, but can't seem to shake off the irrational feeling. For example, feeling like one is going crazy, but rationally knowing that it is not true. Resembles experiencing a bad dream and not being able to wake up.

Forgetfulness - Unable to remember what one ordinarily would remember.

Insomnia - Sleeplessness caused by physical stress, mental stress or stimulants, such as coffee or medications; a condition of being abnormally awake when one would ordinarily be able to fall and remain asleep.

Irritability - An abnormal reaction of being annoyed or disturbed in response to a stimulus in the environment.

Jitteriness - Nervous fidgeting without apparent cause.

Lethargy - Mental and physical sluggishness and *apathy* (a feeling of hopelessness that "nothing can be done") which can deteriorate into an unconscious state resembling deep sleep. A numbed state of mind.

Libido Decreased - An abnormal loss of sexual energy or desire.

Panic Reaction - A sudden, overpowering, chaotic and confused mental state of terror resulting in being doubt-ridden, often accompanied with *hyperventilation* and extreme anxiety.

Restlessness Aggravated - A constantly worsening troubled state of mind characterized by increased nervousness, inability to relax and quick temper.

Somnolence - Feeling sleepy all the time or having a condition of semi-consciousness.

Suicide Attempt - An unsuccessful deliberate attack on one's own life with the intention of ending it.

Suicidal Tendency - Most likely will attempt to kill oneself.

Tremulousness Nervous - Very jumpy, shaky, and uneasy, while feeling fearful and timid. The condition is characterized by dread of the future, involuntary quivering, trembling, and feeling distressed and suddenly upset.

Yawning - Involuntary opening of the mouth with deep inhalation of air.

REPRODUCTIVE FEMALE

Breast Neoplasm - A tumor or cancer, of either of the two milk-secreting organs on the chest of a woman.

Menorrhagia - Abnormally heavy menstrual period or a menstrual flow that has continued for an unusually long period of time.

Menstrual Cramps - Painful, involuntary uterus contractions that women experience around the time of their menstrual period, sometimes causing pain in the lower back and thighs.

Menstrual Disorder - A disturbance or derangement in the normal function of a woman's menstrual period.

Pelvic Inflammation - The reaction of the body to infectious, allergic or chemical irritation, which, in turn, causes tissue irritation, injury, or bacterial infection characterized by pain, redness, swelling, and sometimes loss of function. The reaction usually begins in the uterus and spreads to the fallopian tubes, ovaries and other areas in the hipbone region of the body.

Premenstrual Syndrome - Various physical and mental symptoms commonly experienced by women of childbearing age usually 2 to 7 days before the start of their monthly period. There are over 150 symptoms including eating binges, behavioral changes, moodiness, irritability, fatigue, fluid retention, breast tenderness, headaches, bloating, anxiety and depression. The symptoms cease shortly after the period begins and disappear with menopause.

Spotting Between Menses - Abnormal bleeding between periods. Unusual spotting between menstrual cycles.

RESPIRATORY SYSTEM (ORGANS INVOLVED IN BREATHING)

Asthma - A disease of the breathing system initiated by an allergic reaction or a chemical, with repeated attacks of coughing, sticky mucus, wheezing, shortness of breath and a tight feeling in the chest. The disease can reach a state where it stops a person from exhaling, leading to unconsciousness and death.

Breath Shortness - Unnatural breathing, using a lot of effort resulting in not enough air taken in by the body.

Bronchitis - Inflammation of the two main breathing tubes leading from the windpipe to the lungs. The disease is marked by coughing, a low-grade fever, chest pain and hoarseness. Can also be caused by an allergic reaction.

Coughing - A cough is the response to an irritation, such as mucus, that causes the muscles controlling the breathing process to expel air from the lungs suddenly and noisily to keep the air passages free from the irritating material.

Laryngitis - Inflammation of the voice box characterized by hoarseness, sore throat, and coughing. It can be caused by straining the voice or exposure to infectious, allergic or chemical irritation.

Nasal Congestion - The presence of an abnormal amount of fluid in the nose.

Pneumonia Tracheitis - Bacterial infection of the air passageways and lungs that causes redness, swelling and pain in the windpipe. Other symptoms are high fever, chills, pain in the chest, difficulty breathing and coughing with mucus discharge.

Rhinitis - Chemical irritation causing pain, redness and swelling in the mucus membranes of the nose.

Sinus Congestion - The mucus-lined areas of the bones in the face that are thought to help warm and moisten air to the nose. These areas become clogged with excess fluid or become infected.

Sinus Headache - An abnormal amount of fluid in the hollows of the facial bone structure, especially around the nose. This excess fluid creates pressure, causing pain in the head.

Sinusitis - The body reacting to chemical irritation causing redness, swelling and pain in the area of the hollows in the facial bones especially around the nose.

SKELETAL

Neck/Shoulder Pain - Hurtful sensations of the nerve endings caused by damage to the tissues in the neck and shoulder, signaling danger of disease.

SKIN AND APPENDAGES (SKIN, LEGS AND ARMS)

Acne - Eruptions of the oil glands of the skin, especially on the face, marked by pimples, blackheads, whiteheads, bumps and more severely, by cysts and scarring.

Alopecia - The loss of hair, baldness.

Angioedema - Intense itching and swelling welts on the skin called hives caused by an allergic reaction to internal or external agents. The reaction is common to a food or a drug. Chronic cases can last for a long period of time.

Dermatitis - Generally irritated skin that can be caused by any of a number of irritating conditions, such as parasites, fungus, bacteria, or foreign substances causing an allergic reaction. It is a general in-flammation of the skin.

Dry Lips - The lack of normal moisture in the fleshy folds that surround the mouth.

Dry Skin - The lack of normal moisture/oils in the surface layer of the body. The skin is the body's largest organ.

Epidermal Necrolysis - An abnormal condition in which a large portion of the skin becomes intensely red and peels off like a second-degree burn. Symptoms often include blistering.

Eczema - A severe or continuing skin disease marked by redness, crusting and scaling, with watery blisters and itching. It is often difficult to treat and will sometimes go away only to reappear again.

Folliculitis - Inflammation of a follicle (small body sac), especially a hair follicle. A hair follicle contains the root of a hair.

Furunculosis - Skin boils that show up repeatedly.

Lipoma - A tumor of mostly fat cells that is not health endangering.

Pruritus - Extreme itching of often-undamaged skin.

Rash - A skin eruption or discoloration that may or may not be itching, tingling, burning or painful. It may be caused by an allergy, a skin irritation or a skin disease.

Skin Nodule - A bulge, knob, swelling or outgrowth in the skin that is a mass of tissue or cells.

RELATED TO THE SENSES

Conjunctivitis - Infection of the membrane that covers the eyeball and lines the eyelid, caused by a virus, allergic reaction or an irritating chemical. It is characterized by redness, a discharge of fluid and itching.

Dry Eyes - Not enough moisture in the eyes.

Earache - Pain in the ear.

Eye Infection - The invasion of the eye tissue by a bacteria, virus, fungus, etc, causing damage to the tissue, with toxicity. Infection spreading in the body progresses into disease.

Eye Irritation - An inflammation of the eye.

Metallic Taste - A range of taste impairment from distorted taste to a complete loss of taste.

Pupils Dilated - Abnormal expansion of the black circular opening in the center of the eye.

Taste Alteration - Abnormal flavor detection in food.

Tinnitus - A buzzing, ringing or whistling sound in one or both ears occurring from the use of certain drugs.

Vision Abnormal - Normal images are seen differently by the viewer than by others.

Vision Blurred - Eyesight is dim or indistinct and hazy in outline or appearance.

Visual Disturbance - Eyesight is interfered with or interrupted. Examples of disturbances are light sensitivity and the inability to easily distinguish colors.

URINARY SYSTEM

Blood in Urine - Blood is present when one empties the liquid waste product of the kidneys through the bladder by urinating in the toilet, turning the water pink to bright red. Or spots of blood are observable in the water after urinating.

Dysuria - Difficult or painful urination.

Kidney Stone - Small hard masses of salt deposits that the kidney forms.

Urinary Frequency - Having to urinate more often than usual or between unusually short time periods.

Urinary Tract Infection - An invasion of bacteria, viruses, fungi, etc., of the system in the body. This starts with the kidneys, which eliminate urine from the body. If the invasion goes unchecked, it can injure tissue and progress into disease.

Urinary Urgency - A sudden compelling urge to urinate, accompanied by discomfort in the bladder.

UROGENITAL (URINARY TRACT AND/OR GENITAL STRUCTURES OR FUNCTIONS)

Anorgasmia - Failure to experience an orgasm.

Ejaculation Disorder - Dysfunction of the discharge of semen during orgasm.

Menstrual Disorder - Dysfunction of the discharge during the monthly menstrual cycle.

VIOLENT OR PHYSICALLY DANGEROUS SIDE EFFECTS

Acute Renal Failure - The kidneys stop excreting waste products properly, leading to rapid poisoning (toxicity) in the body.

Anaphylaxis - A violent, sudden, and severe drop in blood pressure caused by a re-exposure to a foreign protein or a second dosage of a drug that may be fatal unless emergency treatment is given right away.

Grand Mal Seizures (or Convulsions) - A recurring sudden, violent and involuntary attack of muscle spasms with a loss of consciousness.

Neuroleptic Malignant Syndrome - A life threatening, rare reaction to an anti-psychotic drug marked by fever, muscular rigidity, changed mental status and dysfunction of the autonomic nervous system.

Pancreatitis - Chemical irritation with redness, swelling and pain in the pancreas where digestive enzymes and hormones are secreted.

QT Prolongation - A very fast heart rhythm disturbance that is too fast for the heart to beat effectively so the blood to the brain falls, causing a sudden loss of consciousness. May cause sudden cardiac arrest.

Rhabdomyolysis - The breakdown and release of muscle fibers into the circulatory system. Some of the fibers are poisonous to the kidney and frequently result in kidney damage.

Serotonin Syndrome - A disorder brought on by excessive levels of *serotonin*. Caused by drugs and can be fatal. Symptoms include euphoria, drowsiness, sustained and rapid eye movement, agitation, reflexes overreacting, rapid muscle contractions, abnormal movements of the foot, clumsiness, feeling drunk and dizzy without any intake of alcohol, jaw muscles contracting and relaxing excessively, muscle twitching, high body temperature, rigid body, rotating mental status - including confusion and excessive happiness - diarrhea and loss of consciousness.

Thrombocytopenia - An abnormal decrease in the number of blood platelets in the circulatory system. A decrease in platelets causes a decrease in the ability of the blood to clot when necessary.

Torsades de Pointes - Unusually rapid heart rhythm starting in the lower heart chambers. If the short bursts of rapid heart rhythm continue for a prolonged period, it can degenerate into a more rapid rhythm and can be fatal.

Benzodiazepine Side Effects

CARDIAC DISORDERS

Palpitation - Perceptible forcible pulsation of the heart, usually with an increase in frequency or force, with or without irregularity in rhythm.

Tachycardia - Rapid heart rate.

EAR AND LABYRINTH DISORDERS

Ear pain - Any pain connected to the inner or outer portion of the ear.

Tinnitus - A sound in one ear or both ears, such as buzzing, ringing, or whistling, occurring without an external stimulus and usually caused by a separate condition, such as the use of benzodiazepines.

Vertigo - A sensation of irregular or whirling motion, either of oneself or of external objects.

EYE DISORDER

Blurred vision - Compared to normal, a distortion of vision.

Mydriasis - Prolonged abnormal dilation of the pupil of the eye induced by a drug or caused by disease.

Photophobia - An abnormal sensitivity to or intolerance of light, especially by the eyes, as may be caused by eye inflammation. An abnormal fear of light.

GASTROINTESTIONAL DISORDERS

Abdominal pain - Pain between the chest and pelvis, stomach, intestines, liver, spleen, and pancreas.

Constipation - Difficulty having normal bowel movement.

Diarrhea - Excessive and frequent evacuation of watery feces.

Dry mouth - When the mouth is dry beyond what might be normal.

Dyspepsia - Disturbed digestion; indigestion.

Dysphagia - Difficulty in swallowing or inability to swallow.

Nausea - A feeling of sickness with the urge to vomit.

Pharyngolaryngeal syndrome - Of or pertaining to the larynx or pharynx.

Salivary hypersecretion - A continual or excessive amount of saliva that is uncontrollable.

Vomiting - Ejecting all or part of the stomach contents.

GENERAL DISORDERS

Asthenia - Loss or lack of bodily strength.

Chest tightness - A feeling in the chest of contraction.

Edema - An accumulation of an excessive amount of watery fluid in cells, tissues, or body cavities.

Fatigue – The body feeling drained of energy

Feeling drunk - Feelings associated with drinking too much alcohol.

Feeling hot or cold - An uncontrollable feeling of being too hot or cold that is abnormal for the temperature.

Feeling jittery - An uneasy feeling often associated with the inability to remain still.

Hangover - Feeling like the day after consuming too much alcohol. All or a few hangover sensations may be present.

Increased energy - An abnormal amount of energy bordering on hyperness.

Loss of control of legs – Inability to control legs, such as restless leg syndrome.

Malaise - A vague feeling of bodily discomfort, as at the beginning of an illness.

Pyrexia - Fever

Rigors - Shivering or trembling, as caused by a chill. A state of rigidity in living tissues or organs that prevents response to stimuli.

Sluggishness - A fatigue type feeling or dull.

Thirst - An abnormal sensation of needing liquid.

Weakness - A reduced state of normal energy and stamina.

INFECTIONS AND INFESTATIONS

Influenza symptoms - The body feeling and at times the manifestation of flue like symptoms.

Upper respiratory tract infections - Infection of the nose, sinuses, pharynx (part of neck and throat) or larynx (commonly known as the voice box).

MENTAL DISORDERS

Abnormal dreams - Nightmares or dreams that are upsetting to the individual.

Aggression - Hostile or destructive behavior or actions.

Agitation - A feeling where something or anything could set a person toward anger or combativeness.

Anger - Uncontrollable and volatile emotion with rage; usually an attempt to stop someone or something.

Anxiety - A state of uneasiness and apprehension, as about future uncertainties. A state of intense apprehension, uncertainty, and fear resulting from the anticipation of a threatening event or situation, often to a degree that normal physical and psychological functioning is disrupted.

Apathy - A feeling of no hope, such as if anything can be done it would not work.

Bradyphrenia - A slowness of the mind.

Confusion - An impaired orientation with respect to time, place or the form of an event.

Depersonalization - A state in which the normal sense of personal identity and reality is lost, characterized by feelings that one's actions and speech cannot be controlled.

Depressed mood - A lowering of the state of mind or emotion compared to what a person normally feels.

Depression - A feeling of no hope.

Derealization - The feeling that things in one's surroundings are strange, unreal, or somehow altered, as seen in schizophrenia.

Disorientation – A loss of sense of direction, position, or relationship with one's surroundings. A temporary or permanent state of confusion regarding place, time or personal identity.

Dysphonia - An emotional state marked by anxiety, depression, and restlessness.

Euphoric mood - A feeling of great happiness or well-being, commonly exaggerated and not necessarily well founded.

Hallucination - False or distorted perception of objects or events with a compelling sense of their reality, usually resulting from a traumatic life event or drugs.

Homicidal ideation - The formation of the idea or having the mental image of murder.

Hypomania - A mild form of mania, characterized by hyperactivity and euphoria.

Impulse control - A sudden pushing or driving force. A sudden wish or urge that prompts an unpremeditated act or feeling; an abrupt inclination.

Insomnia - Chronic inability to fall asleep or remain asleep for an adequate length of time.

Irritability - 1. The capacity to respond to stimuli. 2. Abnormal or excessive sensitivity to stimuli of organism, organ, or body part.

Libido decreased - Sexual desire decreased.

Libido increased - Sexual desire increased.

Logorrhea - Incoherent talkativeness.

Mania - A manifestation of bipolar disorder characterized by profuse and rapidly changing ideas, exaggerated gaiety, and excessive physical activity.

Mood swings - The up and or down movement of emotions that are uncontrollable.

Nervousness - Easily agitated or distressed.

Nightmare - A dream creating intense fear, horror, and distress.

Psychomotor retardation - The retardation of movement and or mental process.

Restlessness - An uneasy feeling of not being able to be where one is located comfortably.

Suicidal ideation - The formation of an idea or mental image of killing one self.

METABOLISM AND NUTRITION DISORDERS

Anorexia - Loss of appetite, usually including a fear of becoming obese or a aversion toward food.

Appetite decreased - A decrease in the feeling one needs food for survival.

Appetite increased - An increase of the desire for food for survival.

MUSCULOSKELETAL AND CONNECTIVE TISSUE DISORDERS

Arthralgia - Severe pain in a joint.

Back pain - An unexplained pain anywhere in the back.

Muscle cramps - Muscle being contracted to the point of discomfort.

Muscle twitching - A rhythmic or irregular involuntary movement of any muscle.

Myalgia - Muscular pain or tenderness, especially when nonspecific.

Pain in limb - Pain in arm or leg.

NERVOUS SYSTEM DISORDERS

Amnesia - The loss or impairment of memory.

Ataxia - Loss of the ability to coordinate muscular movement.

Coordination abnormal - Maintaining balance of the body difficult in comparison to what is normal for the person.

Disturbance in attention - Not able to remain as focused as one was able to in the past.

Dizziness - A disorienting sensation such as faintness, light-headedness, or unsteadiness.

Dysarthria - Difficulty in articulating words due to emotional stress or to paralysis or incoordination of the muscles used in speaking.

Dyskinesia - An impairment in the ability to control movements, characterized by spasmodic or repetitive motions of lack of coordination.

Headache - A continual or time specific duration with pressure or pain within the head.

Hypersomnia - A condition in which one sleeps for an excessively long time but is normal in the waking intervals.

Hypoesthesia - Drowsiness.

Hypotonia - Reduced tension or pressure, as of the intraocular fluid in the eyeball. Relaxation of the arteries.

Memory impairment - Not able to recall an instance from the past as well as before.

Mental impairment - The ability to think and reason diminished.

Paresthesia - A skin sensation, such as burning, prickling, itching, or tingling.

Sedation - An over expression of reduction of anxiety, stress, irritability or excitement.

Seizures - A sudden attack, spasm, or convulsion, as in epilepsy.

Sleep apnea - A temporary cessation of breathing while sleeping.

Sleep talking - Speaking words while asleep.

Somnolence - A state of drowsiness; sleepiness. A condition of semi-consciousness approaching coma.

Stupor - A state of impaired consciousness characterized by a marked diminution in the capacity to react to environmental stimuli.

Syncope - A brief loss of consciousness caused by a sudden fall of blood pressure or failure of cardiac systole, resulting in cerebral anemia.

Tremor - An involuntary trembling movement.

RENAL, THORACIC, AND MEDIASTINAL DISORDERS

Difficulty in micturition - Difficulty with urination or the frequency of.

Urinary frequency - An abnormal frequency of urination.

Urinary incontinence - Involuntary leakage of urine.

REPRODUCTIVE SYSTEM AND BREAST DISORDERS

Dysmenorrhea - A condition marked by painful menstruation.

Premenstrual syndrome - A group of symptoms, including abdominal bloating, breast tenderness, headache, fatigue, irritability, and depression.

Sexual dysfunction - A non-normal, for the individual, behavior or ability to have sex.

RESPIRATORY, THORACIC AND MEDIASTINAL DISORDERS

Choking sensation - A feeling of choking with or without cause.

Dyspnea - Difficulty in breathing, often associated with lung or heart disease and resulting in shortness of breath.

Epistaxis - Nosebleed.

Hyperventilation - Abnormally fast or deep respiration resulting in the loss of carbon dioxide from the blood, thereby causing a decrease in blood pressure and sometimes fainting.

Nasal congestion - A stoppage or restriction of the nasal passage.

Rhinitis - Inflammation of the nasal membranes.

Rhinorrhea - A discharge from the mucous membrane, especially if excessive.

VASCULAR DISORDERS

Hot flashes – A sudden, brief sensation of heat, often over the entire body, caused by a transient dilation of blood vessels of the skin.

Hypotension - Abnormally low arterial blood pressure.

SKIN AND SUBCUTANEOUS TISSUE DISORDERS

Clamminess - Abnormally moist, sticky and cold to the touch.

Pruritus - Severe itching, often of undamaged skin.

Rash - A skin eruption.

Sweating increased - Abnormal increase of perspiration.

Urticaria - A skin condition characterized by welts that itch intensely, caused by an allergic reaction, an infection, or nervous condition.

CHAPTER 5

THINGS TO BE AWARE OF

There are several medical situations you need to be aware of before you start this program. First let me repeat, check with your doctor before starting this program. Medically and physically, do this for your health and safety as you travel though this process.

I understand there could be a problem: possibly your doctor does not support tapering off the medication.

In such a case, check The Road Back website *www.theroadback.org* or call us at 1-866-892-0238. We constantly add to our list of doctors who endorse and use The Road Back Program to help their patients taper off psychiatric medications. You can also find doctors more integrative in their approach to medicine and its application in helping patients heal. These doctors have a broader view of medicine, a greater understanding of how nutritional support relates to the body or would be open to and/or schooled in different healing methods.

This is your journey. Find those who will help you travel the proven successful road laid out for you.

Physical Conditions and Drug Interactions

Many people have contacted me over the years, asking about their activities and/or medications taken and whether they can use these in combination with The Road Back Program. My answer? Check with your doctor about medications and how these could interact with other supplements, vitamins, drugs and so on. Having said that, I know various medical conditions and/or drugs could possibly interfere with this program, including the following:

1. **Blood thinners and heart medication**

   Omega 3 and vitamin E both thin the blood. Taking either of these supplements, in conjunction with a medication that is already thinning your blood, could be contra-indicated, or not advised. This is for your doctor to determine.

2. **Clotting agents**

   Some of the supplements used on The Road Back contain naturally high levels of vitamin K. This vitamin has clotting and healing properties, and as such, could create additional clotting that would not be beneficial. Again, this is for your doctor to determine.

Alternative Therapies

While I have personally seen the results from natural health and healing practices, each has its own purpose and end result. Additionally, I have found they can too often be counterproductive when used in conjunction with The Road Back Program. Any alternative therapy or health practice that recommends additional nutrients, supplements, vitamins, drips, sprays, drinks and methodologies can and do exacerbate, aggravate or make worse, the very sensitive process we are trying to guide you through now.

Due to your psychiatric medications, your system is essentially balanced on the "head of a pin," meaning that your tolerance for *anything* can be, or is, very limited.

The Road Back Program has been researched and developed around very specific parameters, undercutting any other health products. While these other health products might be great in a healthy, balanced body, they often do not mix well with psychiatric medications and your tapering process. Right now you need to slowly and safely taper off your medications. Add other health products back into your daily regime after you have completed this venture. Once completely and safely off these medications, by all means, help yourself.

While on The Road Back Program taking various health products adds one more thing to an already overloaded system. Therefore, I emphatically recommend you evaluate these alternative therapies, practices, nutritional items and restrict them until successfully completing your program.

Specifically, anything that moves medications too rapidly through your body should be avoided.

Remember, "Slow and steady wins the race."

CHAPTER 6

GENERAL PRE-TAPERING AND TAPERING INSTRUCTIONS

Despite apparent redundancy, what I am about to say cannot be said too many times, so bear with me.

As you start your road back, I want your journey to be as successful and as smooth as possible. Therefore, I repeat; *you cannot simply quit your medications cold turkey.*

You must methodically taper off these drugs, giving your body all possible assistance to ensure you fully complete this program and are not driven back onto your prescriptions.

Your program consists of a two-part process: First, the pre-taper, which can be done in one week. If you need more time on the pre-taper go-ahead and spend the time but the final relief may not come until you are reducing the medication or until you are completely off the medication. This is a journey back to you through steady steps that become more and more certain over time.

Once finished with the pre-taper, you will start the actual taper. You will start to reduce the medication while continuing your supplements. The number of medications you are currently taking, and your speed of progress each step along the way, will determine the length of the tapering process.

This chapter is an overview of the pre-tapering and tapering process, and what you will do no matter which drug or drugs you are taking.

These steps are vitally important to your success. Please study them carefully to ensure confidence when beginning your personal program.

The Purpose of the Pre-Taper

Just as in running a marathon, swimming a mile, buying a house, or having a baby, you have to build up to the ultimate goal. The same applies with The Road Back Program. You need to stretch your muscles, get some correct nutrients into your system and know how your daily schedule will change. The Pre Taper will set you up for a smooth reduction off your medications.

The Pre-Taper Goals

- Elimination, or a *drastic* reduction, of all existing side effects caused by the medications.

- Determining which supplements created the positive change.

  When you know the exact supplement that eliminated the side effects, you will know how to eliminate that side effect, if it recurs during the reduction phase of your program.

The reasoning: If a withdrawal side effect begins during the taper, odds are that it was one of the existing side effects you had *before you started your pre-taper*.

An example of the importance of the pre-taper is found in the Introduction to *The Art of War* by Sun Tzu, from Thomas Cleary's translation.

"Plan for what is difficult while it is easy, do what is great while it is small. The most difficult things in the world must be done while they are still easy; the greatest things in the world must be done while they are still small."

Nutritional Supplements

Review the Chapter "Nutritionals Used on The Road Back Program" and make sure you have the nutritional supplements on hand. The day before you start your pre-taper, review which supplements you will be taking the next day, and the times you will be taking them. If you will be carrying the supplements with you during the day, and need to put those quantities into smaller containers, do so. If you know that you have a busy schedule on the day that you will start, or any day following that, prepare by making a note of when you need to take your supplements and how you can arrange to do so. If you do not usually carry water with you, or have it available where you will be, take some with you.

As stated earlier, this program is a work in progress. We constantly research better ways to eliminate side effects and speed up the tapering process. This new edition is required due to recent breakthroughs. Today a person can taper completely off their medication in half the time previously required. The changes to the program are fewer supplements used and a two third reduction in time that it takes to complete the pre-taper. The pre-taper has been able to change from taking twenty-two days to seven days.

Your Daily Journal:

Every day you will keep a written record of your progress in a journal.

You are free to copy the journal found in the next chapter and put together your own, or you can find pre-made journals at The Road

Back website. In your Daily Journal you will note certain information over the course of a 24-hour period. These specific statistics are important because they will help you find your way back to center, if you falter at any point during the program. Before going to bed each night, or during the day as you take each step, write down the following:

- The date.

- The time of all medications you took that day and dosage amount.

- All food and drinks, including coffee, water, alcohol, etc; times you ate or drank, and the amount.

- Rate your own progress as to how you feel.

- Rate your energy, appetite, mood and exercise.

- Include anything that you added or deleted from your daily routine.

Keeping the journal allows you to review changes and determine which changes made positive improvements. However, if a problem occurs, the journal allows you to look back and locate which change may have made a negative impact. Locating such will enable you to quickly fix what changed and get yourself back on track.

For example, you may have increased your supplements and "super foods" too quickly or too much, and now you need to reduce them to the quantity you were taking when you last felt good. Or possibly you felt so good from the pre-taper that you added exercise into your day, which created a negative change. Whatever the case, it could be a small and seemingly insignificant change, or it could be a major change that you did not realize you had made. Using your Daily Journal, you will be able to find your way back. The Daily Journal will act like a positive voice sitting on your shoulder reminding you of what works for you, and what does not.

By noting the exact quantity of each supplement you have taken daily, you will know the positive changes are a direct result of the exact amounts and times you took your supplements.

Recreational Drugs and Alcohol

There might not be a lot to say on this subject that you do not already know. Firstly, either of these items, recreational drugs and/or alcohol, can create or bring on unwanted physical symptoms during your tapering process. Use of either could also cause or contribute to existing problems, mask potential problems, or aggravate problems that already exist. While I have said do not change anything you are doing in your life, this is one area where that adage does not apply. Completing The Road Back Program *is not* about "having your cake and eating it too."

Becoming medication-and-symptom-free is your goal. Give yourself the chance to accomplish your goal.

Do Not Change Anything

Since I just told you to stop taking recreational drugs and alcohol, I might now seem to be contradicting myself, but not so.

For example: If you are already on some form of exercise program, and starting The Road Back Program, you would not stop exercising. It is great for your body, and *your* body is accustom to this routine.

If not on an exercise program, do not suddenly start because it seems like a good idea in combination with the tapering process. Your body is not ready for both of these changes at the same time and there could be hell to pay. However, you can go for a slow, casual walk daily if you wish. That is fine and recommended.

Also note the following:

- Do not start a liver-cleansing process, colon cleanse, etc. and the taper at the same time.

- Do not stop drinking coffee, smoking or abruptly change your diet and start this program at the same time.

Each one of these dos and don'ts: a) has its own chemical response in your system and b) any of these can either speed up or slow down the flow of medication you are taking through your body, and could create withdrawal side effects.

While some supplements are good for you and some supplements may not be as beneficial, it will be too hard to sort out what causes what, therefore you may find it difficult to keep yourself on a steady path gaining momentum and success. You get the point – use your head. Examine the options and choose the one that adheres as closely to The Road Back Program as possible.

Deviation from The Road Back Program

You might think deviating from the program would be obvious and easy to detect. Not always.

The Road Back Program usually works quickly with the person quickly experiencing a vast improvement. This blessing can also be a curse. In the first years of the program, a person would typically feel a major positive change about halfway through the tapering portion. Now they frequently experience major positive change after a few days on the pre-taper. The creation of the supplements and the time of day each is taken have greatly sped up the program. Imagine feeling as though you had never taken a drug only one week after starting the pre-taper part of The Road Back Program.

However, when this major positive change occurs, a person can feel so good that he or she begins doing things they have wanted to do for years, such as quitting smoking, giving up coffee or starting a major exercise program.

Then they suddenly crash and wonder why!

I first experienced this curse in 1999 when a woman called who was tapering off her medication. After first doing well, suddenly she was not. She had tried to taper off an antidepressant medication several times over the years before starting The Road Back Program, never reducing the drug without extreme withdrawal and always returning to her original dosage. This time she had been halfway off her medication and feeling great.

It took two weeks to figure out what changed. I asked every question I could think of; there was something she was doing differently. I finally found out that typically, every six months, she went onto an all-protein diet. This was so "normal" for her she never thought to mention, or view it, as a major change in her lifestyle. However, this diet change hugely impacted her progress, and *was* the major deviation from the program. Once the change was discovered, she re-started her tapering program from square one and successfully completed tapering off the antidepressant.

I cannot over stress looking for and finding obvious as well as subtle changes if you experience a negative change during this program.

Another major deviation from the program can occur – you feel so good, you forget to take your medication(s). This is a no-no, but happens. Lower the medication only at specific amounts and make that gradual reduction. Numerous people over the years have begun a pre-taper while suffering from widely varying side effects. Taking psychiatric medications for years, they had tried to get off the drugs countless times. After beginning the pre-taper and finally sleeping through the night for the first time in months, their daytime anxiety vanished. Three days later, they forgot to take their medication at bedtime. The next day, they went into full withdrawal and began to question whether The Road Back Program was right for them. The only problem was forgetting to take their medication.

These variations or deviations from the program can also be extremely troubling for a doctor. He or she can only help guide you through the steps with all the information on hand. Again, it is imperative that: a) you write everything down in your Daily Journal, including things you might think have no bearing whatsoever, and b) bring your Daily Journal to your doctor visits, so that together you can chart your progress and get back to square one if needed.

"Super Foods"

A deviation from The Road Back Program can also take place with the "super foods" used on the program. Once you feel a positive change with the Power Barley Formula, do not increase it further during the pre-taper.

I often make this joke about Texans and Power Barley Formula. Big, or better yet bigger, is better in Texas. On a trip to Texas I described how to use the Power Barley Formula, what to look for regarding positive changes and to not increase that product once positive change is achieved.

Two weeks later, a Texan called raving about her positive changes. One week later, the same person called again, saying they did not feel as well and were wondering what could have happened. This was not too difficult to solve. Texans and Power Barley Formula? The person had doubled the Power Barley Formula amount that brought on the positive changes. If one teaspoon three times a day made you feel that good, 2 teaspoons 3 times a day should make you feel twice as good, was the thought process.

Once the Texan went back to the right amount for her body, she felt good again.

Major Improvement

The Texan story leads us to the definition of major change - a major improvement. A major improvement is what you are going for with the pre-taper.

If you have extreme daytime anxiety and are able to reduce it to a point where you have to stop and look for anxiety to even see or feel any, you have had a major improvement.

If you could not sleep more than two hours a night and are now able to sleep four to five hours, wake up and then go back to sleep, that is a major improvement.

If every joint in your body ached, and now you have only a little ache in the morning when you awake that goes away within the first few minutes, you have experienced a major improvement.

If you felt a major depression every day and now you feel a little depressed occasionally, you have had a major improvement.

If you feel like you are not even taking a medication now, you have had a major improvement.

Major changes are what you are going for during the pre-taper. The goal is to alleviate major complaints or reduce them to the point of being very acceptable and not in the way of day-to-day life, so that you can fully taper off the medication and "live life."

Once a "super food" or supplement provides relief or a major improvement, there is no need to keep *increasing* that product.

Steady State: The term "steady state" has special definitions in biochemistry, chemistry, electronics and even macroeconomics.

In The Road Back Program "steady state" is defined as: A constant level or a level of action that allows a balance between two or more substances.

A *constant level* would be maintaining a level of a supplement in the body to a degree where it never drops below a certain point. Much like the half-life of medication, keeping enough of a substance in the body at a specific strength gives a result. If you skip a dosage of medication, withdrawal begins. If you skip a serving of a supplement, withdrawal does not take place, but you do lose the steady or constant state of the supplement.

A *level of action that allows a balance between two or more substances* is different from a *constant level*. Psychiatric medications alter hormones and the adrenals. When a "steady state" occurs with the nutritionals at a *constant level*, the cells will use the nutrients to begin working with each other, balancing each other, allowing the cells to receive energy and exchange back to other cells desired substances for optimum survival.

During the pre-taper, one goal is finding the "steady state" of each nutritional for your body. Age, height, weight, gender, how long you have been using a medication or the type of medication you might be using *cannot* be used to predict the correct amount of a nutritional in this program. This takes trial and success.

If You Have Anxiety or Insomnia, What to Expect

The following chart is the result of a double-blind randomized controlled trial of the benzodiazepine Oxazepam compared to the type of passion flower used in this program. Oxazepam is also marketed under the names Alepam, Murelax, Oxascand, Serax, Serepax, Seresta and Sobril.

The trial was for treatment of generalized anxiety.

Two groups were used. One group received Oxazepam plus a placebo while the other used Passion Flower and a placebo. The Body Calm Supreme used with The Road Back Program is the passion flower available that is closest to that used in the trial.

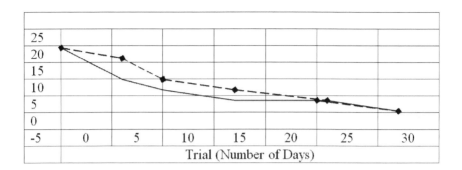

Anxiety Reduction Chart
Oxazepam plus placebo
Passion Flower plus placebo

Left Column is the Hamilton Anxiety Score.

Notice the gradual reduction of anxiety over 30 days. During your pre-taper the anxiety should begin to lessen and the second week should bring a marked decrease of anxiety. Use the graph located after the "Daily Journal" chapter to chart your own progress.

Calcium-Induced Side Effects With Benzodiazepines and Anti-Convulsants

- When taking benzodiazepines and/or anti-convulsants, do not take a supplement containing ionic calcium.

If you are taking an antidepressant or anti-psychotic medication and anxiety is a major complaint, avoid ionic calcium as well.

If you are going to take calcium, make sure to include 5 grams each day of Calsorption to improve the calcium absorption and ideally use a calcium product like CalesiumD.

Ionic calcium and "plain" or unaltered calcium differ in that ionic calcium is altered into a form the body absorbs instantly versus "plain" or unaltered calcium, which breaks down in the body more slowly. An ionic calcium product either dissolves or fizzes when put into hot or cold liquid.

While either type of calcium supplements a natural, healthy diet, do not use ionic calcium if taking a benzodiazepine or if suffering from anxiety. Calcium is something all bodies require, and one main property is assisting with the correct functioning of nerve impulses. While you want your nerves and their impulses functioning correctly at all times, you do not want or need to increase or "feed" this nerve stimulation while you are taking and/or trying to taper off of benzodiazepines and/or anti-convulsants.

Calcium stimulates electrical discharge of the nerves. The stimulation of nerve impulses is the primary problem associated with using ionic calcium along with a benzodiazepine or anticonvulsant.

Clinical trials have shown that blocking calcium can help protect a person from the worst benzodiazepine withdrawal symptoms.

Calcium-induced side effects while taking a benzodiazepine or anti-convulsant can include:

- Hyperkinesia: an abnormal increase in muscular activity, hyperactivity, especially in children.

- Hyperthermia: unusually high body temperature.

- Hyper aggression.

- Audiogenic seizures: Seizures caused by loud sounds and noises.

- Increased anxiety.

- Psychosis.

- Numbness around the mouth.

- Tingling in the extremities.

- Shortness of breath.

It is vital that you ensure you are not taking an ionic calcium supplement while using a benzodiazepine or anti-convulsant.

Several patients and physicians have contacted The Road Back with questions about using calcium as part of The Road Back Program.

Suggestion: If you are taking a calcium supplement and suffer from anxiety, stop the calcium supplement for three days. See if the anxiety goes away or greatly subsides. If the anxiety subsides, there is nothing left to argue about. If the anxiety stays the same, it is not the calcium. Keep taking the calcium!

Your Next Step

- If you are taking a benzodiazepine, anti-convulsant, anti-anxiety or sleep medication, follow the instructions found in the chapter "Pre-Taper for Benzodiazepine, Anti-convulsant, Anti-anxiety, and Sleep Medication" in Chapter 9.

- If you are taking an antidepressant, anti-psychotic or ADHD medication, follow the instructions found in the chapter "Pre-Taper for Antidepressants, Anti-Psychotics, and ADHD Medication" in Chapter 10.

- If you are taking a benzodiazepine, anti-convulsant, anti-anxiety or sleep medication along with an antidepressant, anti-psychotic or ADHD medication follow the instructions found in the chapter "Pre-Taper for Antidepressants, Anti-Psychotics, and ADHD Medication" in Chapter 10. In that chapter, there is a section "If You Have Anxiety or Insomnia." Follow the pre-taper instructions in that section.

Two Key Components for Accomplishing a Complete and Successful Taper:

- Fully complete your *pre-tapering* program before starting your medication- reduction tapering program.

- Taper off the medication using the correct reduction amount to match your body. Slow and gradual will win this race each and every time.

CHAPTER 7

DAILY JOURNAL

Date: _____ Pre-Taper/Taper (Circle one) Day #_____ Step # _____

Note: <u>**Do Not Change Eating or Exercise Habits During The Program!**</u>

Current Drugs & Dosages: (List all taken, time of day and amount)

_____   _____   _____   _____

_____   _____   _____   _____

Food and Liquid:
(List all food and liquid consumed, time of day and amount)

The Road Back Nutritionals: (List all taken, time of day and amount)

<u>Rate the Following Areas Using a Scale of 1 to 10</u>: (Rate daytime anxiety at bedtime and rate the previous night's sleep first thing in the morning. Rate all other items before bedtime.)

Symptom	1-10 Rating	List All Changes Made During the Day
Aches		
Anxiety		
Appetite		
Body Pains		
Energy		
Exercise		
Fatigue		

Mood		
Sleep		

CHAPTER 8

GRAPH YOUR SUCCESS

A graph for each symptom you are rating each day can greatly help tracking your progress and allow you to look back at how far you have come.

See an example below of how to fill in the graph. The next page is a blank graph for you to copy or recreate on your own.

Pre-Taper / Taper (Circle one)   Day # _____ Step # _____

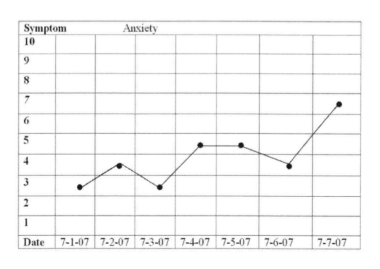

Notice the trend change beginning on the fourth. The trend continues the next day and then drops one day, but rebounds to a 7-rating on the last day of the week.

This is a normal daily trend during the beginning of the pre-taper. If you have already quit taking the medication and are suffering from withdrawal side effects, make sure you use these graphs. I understand you need hope, and seeing for yourself may spark the hope that inspires you to continue and make it back.

After graphing each day and symptom for a period of time, you will see a longer-term trend. Placing each graph side-by-side you can easily see your ratings for several weeks and your trend for each symptom.

Make sure you take your Daily Journal and graphs to your doctor visits.

By running each graph for seven days, you can attach one completed graph to seven days of your Daily Journal and create a weekly file.

Daily Graph

Symptom							
10							
9							
8							
7							
6							
5							
4							
3							
2							
1							
Date							

PRE-TAPER FOR BENZODIAZEPINES, ANTI-ANXIETY, ANTICONVULSANTS AND SLEEP MEDICATION

"I am taking Klonopin. After one week on your program, I do not feel like I am taking a benzo. I am sleeping better than I ever have in my life. Vivid dreams have vanished and if I wake up in the middle of the night, I can go right back to sleep. I will be starting the taper next week and I am very nervous. Every time I have tried to quit in the past, the withdrawal was too much. Everything you have said in your book has been true so far so I probably should not be nervous."

G.Q.
Green Bay, WI.

If you have not yet read the entire chapter "General Pre-Tapering and Tapering Guidelines," please do so before continuing with this chapter. Reading and understanding the "General Pre-Tapering and Tapering Guidelines" is *vital* before starting the pre-taper.

Starting Your Pre-Taper

Note: This pre-taper addresses several types of medication as noted in the chapter title. If the only drug named is a benzodiazepine, please take that to mean the medications (Benzodiazepine, *Antianxiety, Anticonvulsant and Sleep Medication*).

Physically, during the pre-taper and taper, you need to address the immune system, and what is called the pituitary adrenal-axis, along with other enzymes that regulate anxiety and sleep. What may be physical, but is viewed more as mental, will be anxiety, insomnia and other symptoms of how you feel subjectively.

You will begin your pre-taper by taking JNK supplement, Body Calm and Body Calm Supreme. These three supplements should take care of most or all daytime anxiety, panic attacks and sleep problems. If you have taken a benzodiazepine for a prolonged period and you have depression or a tingling or numbness of the extremities, the JNK supplement will be vital. The JNK supplement includes the vitamin biotin in the formula and prolonged use of a benzodiazepine will deplete biotin massively and lead to depression and the tingling or numbness.

You may have side effects other than anxiety and insomnia that are your main concern. While not addressed specifically in this text, those side effects will usually respond to the pre-taper as well. Review the optional supplements available with this program if side effects are not going away completely.

Remember, as soon as you start the pre-taper, you simultaneously begin keeping your Daily Journal.

- *Make sure to note when existing side effects stop or when there is a major improvement. This is very important.*

You will then know which supplement turns off which side effect(s) or caused the major improvement. You will need to know this to successfully complete both the pre-taper and the full taper. The pre-taper addresses the normal cycle of anxiety/insomnia/anxiety associated with benzodiazepines.

Anxiety both first thing in the morning and again in the afternoon are *very* common side effects of benzodiazepines, anti-anxiety, anticonvulsant and sleep medications. When using these medications, by the time you are ready to go to sleep at night you are too stressed out and fatigued from dealing with anxiety difficulties all day long. Sleep simply may not happen, and you could easily end up feeling depressed due to this continuing cycle of anxiety, no sleep, anxiety, no sleep – endlessly.

If you are also experiencing some degree of depression, do not be surprised if the depression lifts during the pre-taper as your ability to sleep improves or the daytime anxiety abates. But, even as you start to experience relief from your symptoms, *do not change anything*; just continue with the program. There are still many, many gains available as you move through and complete The Road Back Program.

Pre-Taper Goal:

- Improved sleep.

- Vast reduction or elimination of anxiety and insomnia.

- Lessening or elimination of other medication-induced side effects.

Supplements you will take:

- Body Calm.

- Body Calm Supreme.

- JNK

Day One:

Action:

- Rate your daytime anxiety, panic attacks, insomnia and other side effects. Use the Daily Journal and rate anxiety, sleep and any additional symptoms you may be experiencing from 1 to 10. Rate with number 1 being the worst and number 10 being no side effect or symptom remaining.

- Rate the previous night's sleep first thing the next morning.

- Rate the daytime anxiety just before bedtime of that day.

If you take your medication first thing in the morning, take the medication as normal and 1 hour later take the morning supplements.

Morning Supplement:

JNK – Take 1 packet in the morning.

Body Calm: 1 capsule.

Throughout the rest of the day, alternate the Body Calm and Body Calm Supreme every 2 hours. Your morning would start out with the Body Calm capsule and two hours later you would take a Body Calm Supreme capsule.

If you find the Body Calm Supreme makes you tired during the daytime, replace it with the Body Calm and just use the Body Calm Supreme at bedtime.

You can use 2 Body Calm capsules every two hours during the daytime if you wish and up to three capsules of Body Calm Supreme at bedtime if needed for a restful sleep.

Usually, the anxiety will come and go at the same time of the day. If anxiety usually returns or increases at noon, take the Body

Calm at 11:30 am each day or if the anxiety always comes back stronger at 1 pm, make sure to take the Body Calm at noon each day. You can adjust when and how much Body Calm you take according to the time and severity of the anxiety.

Each person does not respond the same to the Body Calm and Body Calm Supreme. Some people prefer to take the Body Calm Supreme every 2 hours during the daytime, while others prefer the Body Calm every 2 hours. Use this first week to find what is best for you.

Bedtime:

Body Calm Supreme: 1 capsule (up to 3 if needed)

After seven full days of the pre-taper, you are ready to move to the tapering portion of the program. Proceed to the chapter How to Taper Off Benzodiazepines, Anti-anxiety and Sleep Medications.

You can also call our support line, 1-866-892-0238 or send an e-mail to info@theroadback.org, for free support and guidance. Please use us; you do not have to do this alone.

CHAPTER *10*

PRE-TAPER FOR ANTIDEPRESSANTS, ANTIPSYCHOTICS, AND ADHD MEDICATIONS

(Abilify, Adderall, Anafranil, Adapin, Celexa, Concerta, Cymbalta, Effexor, Elavil, Haldol, Lexapro, Luvox, Paxil, Prozac, Remeron, Risperdal, Ritalin, Seroquel, Serzone, Strattera, Thorazine, Wellbutrin, Zoloft, Zyprexa etc.)

"I am doing great on the Taper Program. I have successfully gotten off Elavil. I had been on it for about 10 years. I have tried in the past to go off cold turkey and I got so sick each time that I had to go back to it. I finally realized it wasn't the new medications making me sick. It was withdrawal from Elavil. (No doctor recognized my symptoms as withdrawal and I went to 3 different ones trying to get off of it and onto something with fewer side effects.) I have followed the program as indicated and have had no withdrawal effects. I am amazed. I have been completely off for 10 days now. Thank you for making this solution known to the general public."

"I made the mistake and quit my antidepressant cold turkey. The side effects were nausea, constant headache, anxiety, no sleep, that brain zap and a whirling in my head. James, your assistance, and guiding me through the first days has made all the difference. Nausea is gone, headache is gone, brain zaps quit within one hour like you said, and the remaining side effects are so small I can deal with them. I do not know how I can ever repay you for saving my life. Unless someone has been through this, they may not know what I am talking about."

"I am like many others. I decided to come off Prozac by myself in one week. Long story short, you saved my life. Deepest gratitude."

"I am officially off of all SSRIs. I have been "drug free" since Saturday and so far I feel great. This is the longest I have gone without taking either Paxil or Celexa in about four years and I have no regrets!"

If you have not read the entire chapter "General Pre-Tapering and Tapering Instructions," please do so before continuing with this chapter. Reading and understanding the chapter "General Pre-Tapering and Tapering Instructions" is vital before starting the pre-taper.

Antipsychotic and Mood Stabilizer Medications

Make sure to read the section about these medications on page 95.

Starting Your Pre-Taper

This pre-taper is divided into two separate pre-taper programs to accommodate the side effects you currently experience.

- If you are suffering from anxiety and insomnia, use the Anxiety Insomnia Pre-taper.
- If you do not have anxiety and insomnia, move to the section in this chapter, Fatigue Pre-taper.
- If you feel like you have anxiety, insomnia and fatigue, use the anxiety pre-taper.
- If you do not have anxiety, insomnia or fatigue, use the Fatigue Pre-taper.

PRE-TAPER PROGRAM IF YOU HAVE DAYTIME ANXIETY, AGITATION OR INSOMNIA

As you are experiencing either anxiety during the day and/or insomnia at night as side effects, your pre-taper will include Body Calm, Body Calm Supreme, Omega 3 Supreme, JNK supplement and vitamin E; products specifically used to help relieve these symptoms as well as unwanted head symptoms common with antidepressant withdrawal.

With either anxiety or insomnia present, there are sure to be other symptoms being caused by the daily anxiety and lack of sleep at night. The pre-taper is designed to address the other side effects as well.

Remember, as soon as you start the pre-taper, you will simultaneously start keeping track of your days in the Daily Journal.

Make sure to note when existing side effects stop or when there is a major improvement. This is very important.

You will then know which supplement turns off which side effect(s) or caused the major improvement. You will need to know this in order to complete both the pre-taper and the full taper successfully. The pre-taper is designed to address the normal cycle of anxiety/insomnia/anxiety that takes place.

Anxiety first thing in the morning and a return of the anxiety in the afternoon are both *very* common side effects.

If you are also experiencing some degree of depression, do not be surprised if it goes away during the pre-taper, as your ability to sleep improves or the daytime anxiety abates. But, as you start to experience relief from your symptoms, *do not change anything*; just continue with the program. There are still many, many gains to be had as you move through to full completion of the program.

If you have tried to taper off an antidepressant in the past and experienced head symptoms, which may have included a feeling of an electrical jolt running from the base of the neck to the base of your skull, the omega 3 fish oil should handle that symptom if it is present now and eliminate it from starting during the pre-taper.

If you have nausea or flu-like symptoms, try drinking a few cups of ginger tea each day. Drinking the ginger tea usually helps rather quickly.

Goal:

- Improved sleep.

- A vast reduction or elimination of anxiety and insomnia.

- A lessening or elimination of other medication induced side effects.

Supplements you will take:

- Body Calm.

- Body Calm Supreme.

- JNK

- Omega 3 Supreme.

- Vitamin E

Day One:

Action:

- Rate your daytime anxiety, panic attacks, insomnia and other side effects. Use the Daily Journal and rate anxiety, sleep and any additional symptoms you may be experiencing from 1 to 10. Rate with number 1 being the worst and number 10 being no side effect or symptom remaining.

Take: Body Calm Supreme capsule: 1 capsule.

Time: At bedtime.

If you take medication right at bedtime, take the Body Calm Supreme 1 hour before the medication.

Day Two, Three, Four:

Action:

- Rate your daytime anxiety, panic attacks, insomnia and other side effects. Use the Daily Journal and rate anxiety, sleep and any additional symptoms you may be experiencing from 1 to 10. Rate with number 1 being the worst and number 10 being no side effect or symptom remaining.

- Rate the previous night's sleep first thing the next morning.

- Rate the daytime anxiety just before bedtime of that day.

If you take your medication first thing in the morning, take the medication as normal and 1 hour later take the morning supplements.

Morning Supplements:

Body Calm: 1 capsule.

JNK: Take 1 packet in the morning.

Omega 3 Supreme: 2 softgels.

Vitamin E: 1 softgel

Throughout the rest of the day, take 1 Body Calm capsule every 2 to 4 hours. You will need to adjust the Body Calm to the amount that fits your needs. Some people do fine with 1 capsule every 4 hours for daytime anxiety, while others may need 1 capsule every 2 hours. You can also take 2 capsules of Body Calm at the same time for the desired effect if needed.

Usually, the anxiety will come and go at the same time of the day. If anxiety usually returns or increases at noon, take the Body Calm at 11:30 am each day or if the anxiety always comes back stronger at 1 pm, make sure to take the Body Calm at noon each day. You can adjust when and how much Body Calm you take according to the time and severity of the anxiety.

Some people will respond better to the Body Calm Supreme during the daytime. You can try alternating the Body Calm and Body Calm Supreme every 2 to 4 hours. A few people may respond best with only Body Calm Supreme during the daytime.

Use the pre-taper to find what works best for you with the Body Calm and Body Calm Supreme.

Noon Supplements:

Omega 3 Supreme: 2 softgels

Bedtime:

Body Calm Supreme: 1 capsule

Adjustments you can make with the Body Calm and Body Calm Supreme:

- You can replace the Body Calm with the Body Calm Supreme during the daytime if you need further help with daytime anxiety.

- You can increase the Body Calm Supreme to 3 capsules at bedtime if needed.

Day Five, Six, Seven:

Increase the morning and noon Omega 3 Supreme up to 3 softgels.

Antipsychotic and Mood Stabilizer Medications

The JNK supplement packet is essential if you are taking these medications. Take 1 packet of the JNK first thing in the morning.

Additionally, the supplement CalesiumD should be of great benefit as well. CalesiumD is made from calcium citrate, magnesium and a trace of vitamin D3. A simple calcium supplement, but powerful when used with this program. Take 1 capsule in the morning, 1 more at noon and 1 more capsule around 8 pm.

Take the Body Calm, Omega 3 Supreme and Body Calm Supreme as outlined earlier in this chapter.

After 7 full days of the pre-taper, you are ready to move to the tapering portion of the program. Proceed to the chapter How to Taper Off Antidepressants, Antipsychotics and ADHD Medication.

PRE-TAPER PROGRAM IF YOU HAVE FATIGUE and DO NOT HAVE ANXIETY OR INSOMNIA

Supplements you will take:

- Power Barley Formula

- Omega 3 Supreme

- Vitamin E

- **You can replace the Power Barley Formula with the JNK supplement if you are gluten intolerant or if you also need to lose weight, but make sure to include the JNK Liquid Booster.**

Special Note: You will be increasing the Power Barley Formula slowly over a number of days. The word "Power" in the name is intentional. This barley formula is powerful and unlike any other barley product.

At any time during the pre-taper, when you feel increased energy, a new brightness about yourself, an overall good feeling, DO NOT INCREASE THE POWER BARLEY FORMULA FURTHER.

Day One:

Action:

- Rate fatigue, anxiety, sleep and all side effects. Use the Daily Journal and rate your fatigue, mood, anxiety, sleep and other additional symptoms you may be experiencing from 1 to 10. Rate with number 1 being the worst and number 10 being no side effect or symptom remaining.

If you take medication first thing in the morning, take the medication as usual, wait 1 hour and then take the morning supplements.

Morning supplements:
Power Barley Formula: 1 scoop mixed in water
Omega 3 Supreme: 3 softgels
Vitamin E: 1 softgel

Noon supplements:
Power Barley Formula: 1 scoop mixed in water
Omega 3 Supreme: 3 softgels

Take 1 additional scoop of Power Barley Formula if additional energy is needed later in the day but do not take the Power Barley Formula after 6 pm.

If the noon barley is too much for you, skip the noon barley and try taking your second scoop of the day later in the afternoon.

How to Increase the Power Barley Formula:

You can increase the Power Barley Formula by 1 teaspoon with each serving until you feel your energy increase. It is very important you do not increase the Power Barley Formula more once you feel the first positive change with your fatigue. If you increase it too much you may experience headaches or other detoxification effects. If this happens, just reduce the barley back to the amount you were taking and all symptoms should go away.

You may need to increase the Power Barley Formula up to 1 tablespoon with each serving to handle the fatigue. If so, once the fatigue lifts for 3 full days, try reducing the barley back down again.

Head Symptoms

Many of you starting this program have already reduced your medication or abruptly stopped taking your medication and side effects in the head are severe. If taking 3 of the omega 3 fish oil in the morning and noon did not give you relief, increase the omega 3 fish oil to 4 softgels in the morning and 4 softgels at noon. Fish oil should be the supplement that is able to give you the relief from head symptoms.

If you have insisted on taking a brand of omega 3, other than Omega 3 Supreme from TRB Health, it is time for you to make the change.

After you have been on the pre-taper for seven full days, you are ready to taper the medication. Proceed to the chapter How to Taper off Antidepressants, Antipsychotics and ADHD Medications.

Timed Released or Extended Release Medications

Prepare for your tapering of the medication during the pre-taper. You will need to crossover to a non-time release form of the drug. Timed release drugs only come in dosages with large gaps between dosage amounts and this does not accommodate a gradual reduction.

You will need to get with your pharmacist and doctor and possibly even switch to a generic form of the drug if needed to compound the drug for a gradual reduction. When you crossover to the non-time release, count the crossover as a reduction and do not reduce the drug again for 14-days.

Ideally, you would do the crossover first and not wait until you are at the lowest dosage of the time release drug.

CHAPTER 11

HOW TO TAPER OFF BENZODIAZEPINES, ANTI-ANXIETY, ANTICONVULSANTS AND SLEEP MEDICATIONS

Now that you have completed your pre-taper program, you are ready to start the reduction of your medication.

As incredible as it might seem, this step is the *easy* part of The Road Back Program.

This tapering is slow and gradual. Please do not be let down because I use the word slow. Most people have been trying to get off their medication for months, if not years, and they had no hope in sight before finding this program.

You will also find within the drug manufacturers drug description, a statement suggesting you gradually reduce the medication.

The Taper

If you have tried to taper off these medications before and suffered withdrawal side effects, definitely start the taper slowly. Successfully lower the medication by 2% every 14 days for three reductions, and then try increasing the reduction by 5% every 14 days. If all goes well for you, then continue with the 5% reduction every 14 days. If the 5% reduction makes withdrawal side effects begin and they are unbearable, move back to the 2% reduction and continue at that pace for the rest of the taper.

Make sure you work with the prescribing physician before changing the dosage of your medication.

Ask your physician to write a prescription to accommodate a 2% reduction. Use a compounding pharmacy to fill this prescription. Compounding pharmacies exist all over the country. You can look in your local phone book to search for a compounding pharmacy near you or use the Internet.

If the medication you are taking is a time release or called a sustained release drug, you will need to switch to a form of the medication that allows for an exact and slow reduction. When you make this change-over, count that change as a reduction and do not reduce the dosage until 14 days have passed.

Important Points for Tapering

- Only reduce the medication 2% every *fourteen days for the first three reductions*. The 2% reduction is based on the original dosage of the medication. The 2% reduction is based on milligrams.

- Never skip any days of taking the medication.

- Always take your medication at the same time each day.

- If you take your medication more than once each day, make sure the *total* reduction of the medication is no more than 2%. It would NOT be a reduction of 2% of each dosage taken during the day. If you are reducing by 5% make sure the total reduced during the day is no more than 5%.

- Take each supplement at least half an hour apart from the drug, but ideally, 1 hour apart. It is much better to take the supplements 1 hour after taking the drug, instead of before the drug.

- Continue with your supplements at the same times and amounts established during the pre-taper.

- Continue taking your supplements at least 45 days after you take the last dosage of your medication.

- Remember to fill out your Daily Journal each day and keep taking all the supplements exactly as you did at the end of the pre-taper.

After 3 full reductions at the 2% reduction rate you can increase the taper to a 5% percent reduction of the medication every fourteen days.

Some people and physicians feel this method is too slow. Try reducing faster if you wish, but keep in mind, if the withdrawal is too severe you just need to get stable again and reduce at the speed suggested in this book.

If Withdrawal Side Effects Turn On During the Taper:

Do not reduce the medication again until the symptom goes away. This usually takes a few days or less, and then you can resume the taper.

Do not start making wholesale changes to your daily routine.

If you are having anxiety or insomnia that will not go away and you have tried adjusting the Body Calm and Body Calm Supreme as described in the pre-taper, this would be the time to use the Essential Protein Formula and biotin.

- Take 1 scoop of Essential Protein Formula every 2 hours during the daytime and 2 scoops at bedtime.
- If you are having depression or a feeling that depression is starting, take 5,000 mcg of biotin in the morning and 5,000 mcg of biotin around noon.

Sometimes, increasing a supplement the day before you reduce the medication will be all that is needed. If you are taking 1 Body Calm every 2 hours during the daytime, the day before lowering the medication, increase the Body Calm up to 2 capsules every 2 hours. Stay at that level for 3 days and then reduce the Body Calm back down to 1 every 2 hours again. The same can be done with the Body Calm Supreme during the daytime or at bedtime for sleep.

If these options do not stop the side effects, you will need to go back up to the last dosage of the medication before the side effects started, stay at that level for 14 days and then begin reducing the medication again, but at a reduced amount from there forward.
If you were reducing at 5% and that is when the side effects started, go back to reducing by 2% again.

Tapering off the medication can be this simple. If you have any questions, feel free to contact us at 1-866-892-0238 or info@theroadback.org.

Once you are completely off the medication, follow the chapter Once Off All Medication.

CHAPTER 12

HOW TO TAPER OFF ANTIDEPRESSANTS, ANTIPSYCHOTICS AND ADHD MEDICATION

Having completed your pre-taper program, you are now ready to start reducing your medication. Though not knowing what you may have experienced personally, I do know that the vast majority of people ready for this step feel trepidation because of terrible side effects experienced when they have tried to quit before.

You might have experienced the "electrical zaps" in the head that are very common with stopping antidepressants, a return of depression, anxiety, fatigue, extreme aches and pains or even wound up in a mental hospital.

Incredible as this might seem, this step should be the *easy* part of The Road Back Program.

Note: If you are taking Cogentin along with another medication, you will need to rotate the reduction of the Cogentin and the other medication.

Example: If you are taking Cogentin and Haldol, reduce the Haldol first, wait 14 days and then reduce the Cogentin, wait 14 days and then reduce the Haldol once again, wait 14 days and then reduce the Cogentin again. Repeat this process until off both medications. Reduce the Haldol and Cogentin by the same percentage with each reduction.

The Taper

Successfully reduce the medication by 5% every 14 days for three reductions – then increase the reduction amount to 10% every 14 days throughout the rest of the taper.

People have told me that the 10% reduction every 14 days is far too slow. When I responded, "How long have you been trying to get off the medication?" the answer was usually a few years without success. This is where *slow and steady* wins the race every time.

Again, if you had a problem in the past with tapering off the medication, use the 5% reduction schedule first, have some success and then move to the 10% reduction. Successfully reduce the medication at least 3 times, see for yourself that you can do this and still feel well, and then you and your physician should decide if you should reduce the medication at a larger reduction.

Make sure you work with the prescribing physician before changing the dosage of your medication.

If you are taking a medication that is time release or called extended release, you will need to switch over to the non-time release tablet or liquid. When you switch over, count the switch as a reduction and do not begin to lower the dosage for 14 days after the change is made.

Important Points of the Taper

- Ask your physician to write a prescription to accommodate a 5% reduction. You will need to use a compounding pharmacy to fill this prescription.

- Never skip any days taking your medication.

- Always take your medication at the same time each day.

- If you take your medication more than once each day, make sure the *total* reduction of the medication is no more than 5% or the 10% reduction during the last part of the taper.

- Take each supplement at least half an hour apart from the drug, but ideally, 1 hour apart. It is much better to take the supplements 1 hour after taking the drug, instead of before the drug.

- Continue with your supplements at the same times and amounts established during the pre-taper.

- Take each supplement at the same time each day.

- Continue taking your supplements at least 45 days after you take the last dosage of your medication.

- Remember fill out your Daily Journal each day and keep taking all of the supplements exactly as you were at the end of the pre-taper.

Taper Procedure:

1. Keep taking all supplements exactly as you did at the end of the pre-taper throughout the taper process.

2. Keep your Daily Journal up to date each day.

3. Compound medication.

4. Reduce medication by 5% every 14 days, at least during the first 3 reductions.

5. Only reduce the medication every 14 days.

6. Make sure you have at least 7 consecutive days of feeling very well before reducing the medication again. If this requires you to reduce the medication every 21 days, do that.

7. Never skip any days of taking medication.

8. After 3 successful reductions at 5% and fourteen days have passed begin reducing by 10% every 14 days.

Tapering can be this simple.

What to Do If Side Effects Begin

Withdrawal side effects can happen, but addressing them early and knowing what to do will usually keep them mild and short-lived.

Antidepressant "Electrical Brain Zaps"

The "electrical brain zaps" tend to occur when an antidepressant is reduced. If you are tapering off an antidepressant and begin to get the "brain zaps" (electrical jolt that tends to run from the base of the neck to the base of the skull) address them by doing the following:

a. Start taking 5 Omega 3 Supreme in the morning and 5 at noon.

b. Make sure you are taking 400 i.u. of vitamin E in the morning.

It is important to handle the "brain zaps" fully. If the above steps do not handle the "brain zaps" you should start taking the B vitamin biotin. Biotin helps the body assimilate fatty acids and the fatty acids found in Omega 3 are ultimately the best chance of handling the "brain zaps."

Usually, the side effect will subside the same day or the next day with the increase of the Omega 3 Supreme.

If the head side effect remains mild, but is still present, continue taking the 5 softgels of Omega 3 Supreme until the symptom abates and then return to your previous amount of Ultimate Omega 3. Wait 7 full days and then continue with the taper.

If the head side effects are severe and you find it difficult to function in life due to the pain of the symptom, go back to the last dosage of the antidepressant before this reduction and remain there for 14 days. Going back to the last dosage should get rid of the "electrical zaps" quickly.

The next time you reduce the antidepressant and each reduction thereafter, increase the Omega 3 Supreme to 5 softgels in the morning and 5 softgels at noon 2 days before you reduce the medication, and remain at this level for 5 days after reducing the medication. This approach should avert the occurrence of the "electrical zaps."

If the "electrical zaps" continue with this approach, you will need to lower the medication more slowly. Talk to your physician and get your pharmacist to find a way to fill the prescription to allow for a more gradual reduction. This will handle the taper for you.

Antipsychotic Drugs

Antipsychotic tapering side effects can include psychosis, hearing voices, seeing things that are not there or episodes of extreme aggression.

Increasing the Body Calm Supreme has proven to be effective for these side effects.

- Increase the Body Calm Supreme to 1 capsule every 2 hours during the daytime and up to 3 capsules at bedtime for sleep. Usually increasing the Body Calm Supreme to 1 capsule every 2 hours during the day and up to 3 capsules at bedtime for sleep will help with side effects.

- Sometimes your glucose levels may need to be addressed quickly. If you begin to crave sweets, start the Essential Protein Formula during the daytime by taking 1 scoop every 2 hours with the Body Calm Supreme and take 4 scoops at bedtime. This may take 1 or 2 weeks to handle the cravings.

- If bipolar or schizophrenic, the JNK supplement is essential. If you have not started the JNK and you are not feeling a very positive change, you do need to start the JNK supplement.

- Review your Daily Journal and look for changes you might have made to your routine. If you located a change, go back to exactly what you were doing before the change and all should shortly be well. Allow 7 days for the withdrawal side effect to go away.

Once you are off the medication, make sure you keep taking the supplements for 45 days.

Read the chapter, "Once Off All Medication" and follow the ending program completely.

CHAPTER 13

ONCE OFF ALL MEDICATION

Congratulations! If anyone ever deserved a celebration party for an accomplishment, it is you. You not only made it off your medication, but also adhered to a schedule most other people have never had to confront. Only you can know what I mean.

As stated earlier in this book, you should continue taking all supplements for 45 days after the last dosage of the medication. It takes about 20 days for the enzymes used to metabolize the medication to return to a normal state, and depending on your own DNA, about 19 days for the medication to fully clear your body.

Continue writing in your Daily Journal during this ending of the program.

The supplements used during the program are not addictive and there is no withdrawal from these natural products. However, if you were lacking the nutrients found in a specific supplement and you discontinue using it, you may feel a letdown or a negative change. This would be the same feeling any person would have, even if they have never used these medications.

Omega 3 is needed in our diet. The human body needs an adequate amount of vitamins, minerals, and amino acids from a food source to work at an optimum level. If there were one supplement you would continue taking after the 45-days have passed, it would be omega 3 fish oil.

Once off all medication for 45 days, it is advisable to get a complete physical exam with specific attention to hormones, adrenals, your immune system and insulin/glucose: an all-natural treatment, by a healthcare provider who fully understands that this intricate system is needed.

I strongly urge you to keep taking the JNK supplement you have used during the program for the full 45-days after the last dosage of your medication. The JNK gene needs to be held in check for the body to have time to heal.

Phase Two Detoxification

You have completed a Phase 1 detoxification by tapering off your medication. Drug toxins will still remain in the body tissue, body fats and possible muscle. Removing the remaining toxins is called a Phase 2 Detox.

The recommended procedure to use for a Phase 2 Detox is found in the book, Detox or Die, by Dr. Sherry Rogers M.D. If you need assistance in locating a facility using this detoxification method, call us at 1-866-892-0238 and we will give you a current list of facilities.

Please do not take this part of recovery lightly. Environmental toxins may very well have played a role in why you went on the medication initially and a complete recovery after psychoactive medication usage will be determined on the final removal of their lodged toxins still found in the body.

What to Do With Supplements

After you are off the medication for around 20 days, you may need to begin reducing some of the supplements.

Body Calm and Body Calm Supreme – If you begin to feel tired during the daytime, it may be time to lower the amount of *Body Calm or Body Calm Supreme* used during the daytime.

If you are going to lower either of these supplements during the daytime, lower the Body Calm first. Reduce slowly until the tiredness goes away. Keep your Daily Journal filled out each day. If the tiredness goes away by reducing or eliminating the daytime use of the Body Calm, keep taking the Body Calm Supreme exactly as you have been.

If tiredness persists, take the Body Calm Supreme every 6 hours, instead of every 4 hours during the daytime.

Another option is to begin taking or increasing the amount of Power Barley Formula during the daytime for tiredness.

If you were not able to take the Power Barley Formula during the pre-taper or were only able to take less than the highest amount indicated during the pre-taper, increase the Power Barley Formula instead of lowering the Body Calm or Body Calm Supreme.

Go back to the pre-taper chapter that applies to the medication you were taking and increase the Power Barley Formula as outlined in that chapter. Remember, this is powerful barley, only increase it until the positive change takes place. Continue with the Power Barley until you have finished at least one complete container.

Omega 3 Supreme – If you are taking 4 of the Omega 3 in the morning and at noon, you can reduce the Omega 3 down to 3 softgels in the morning and 3 softgels around noon.

If any head symptoms reappear, increase the Omega 3 back up.

Essential Protein Formula – Continue taking the Essential Protein Formula as you did during the pre-taper and taper process for 45 days.

Power Barley Formula – Keep taking the amount established during the pre-taper for the entire 45 days unless you begin to feel anxiety during the daytime. If you begin to feel anxiety during the daytime, decrease the Power Barley Formula by the same amounts it was increased during the pre-taper. Just reverse the process.

Vitamin E – Continue taking the 400 i.u. of vitamin E for the entire 45-days.

Once again, congratulations on completing The Road Back Program and may your journey in life from this point forward be ever-expanding.

CHAPTER 14

WHAT TO DO IF YOU HAVE ALREADY STARTED TO TAPER OFF YOUR MEDICATION OR QUIT COLD TURKEY

The key to handling withdrawal side effects when you begin to reduce the medication is: **Put Control Back in the Process Again.**

Roughly 80% of the people who begin The Road Back Program have already started to taper off their medication or have gone off their medication abruptly and are experiencing withdrawal side effects. The recommendations or suggestions offered in this chapter come from years of experience assisting these individuals.

First, it is not YOU. That may be difficult to grasp at first, but in time, you will come to understand it was not you; it was the withdrawal side effect.

Immediately do the following if you have abruptly stopped your medication or are reducing the medication and you are having withdrawal side effects:

- Inform the prescribing physician

- Go to the pre-taper chapter in this book that covers your medication.
  Benzodiazepines, anti-anxiety and sleep medications, chapter 9.
  Antidepressants, anti-psychotics and ADHD medications, chapter 10.
- Start the supplements in the pre-taper immediately (Go to www.trbhealth.com or call TRB Health at 1-866-810-3809 for the needed supplements)
- If you are or were taking an antidepressant and you have head symptoms or an electrical jolt type of sensation, go to any store that sells vitamins and purchase a bottle of omega 3 fish oil. Look at the back label of the bottle with the highest amount of EPA content. This should get you some relief quickly, but make sure you get the Omega 3 Supreme from TRB Health for a complete handling.

Relief should come shortly after you start the pre-taper supplements. I understand you may have already quit the medication and you are not actually doing a pre-taper now. Just start taking the supplements as described in the pre-taper and follow the directions as outlined in that chapter.

Medication Decisions

You need to make a decision rather quickly about the medication. I understand some of you absolutely refuse to go back on the medication or to go back up in dosage, but I still need to give you my viewpoint. This is only my viewpoint and should not be taken as medical advice.

1. If you have gone off the drug cold turkey and it has been more than one week since you stopped the drug, going back on the drug is not going to help. It will probably

compound the situation. Start the pre-taper supplements and continue taking them for 45-days after you feel well again. Use the supplements based on the drug you were taking.

2. If it has been less than one week since you stopped the drug cold turkey, go back on the drug to the last dosage you were doing your best at, and do the pre-taper for that type of medication and gradually reduce the drug from that point. You may feel this approach moves you backwards but it should get you off the drug and feeling well once again.

3. If you are reducing the medication and you are experiencing withdrawal side effects, you need to determine the severity of the side effects. If the side effects are too strong, go back up to the last dosage when you were doing better. Start the pre-taper, get stable again and then gradually reduce the medication.

4. If the side effects are on the mild side, quit reducing for now, start the pre-taper for the drug you are taking, after using the supplements for 7-days of the pre-taper, continue with the taper and supplements.

There is really no need to expand on this further. You may feel like death warmed over, but the options are few and they are basic. Keep in mind, how you feel is the drug and that it is not you. Make sure to inform your physician of any choice you make.

Do not give up hope.

CHAPTER 15

HOW TO TAPER OFF
MULTIPLE MEDICATIONS

"Thank you! Thank you! Thank you! I feel 100% better!!!! Oh My Gosh. I cannot believe how great I feel. I'm actually getting ME back. I can see my personality, my spunk, my spark increase gradually each and every day, more and more. I cannot thank you enough. This has changed my life dramatically!

Please let me know how I can help to talk with others, to educate them, encourage them on getting their lives back and not depending on these drugs.

I know I still have a long way before I am completely healed. I look at it like this, though. If I feel this great now and I've only been off these 2 drugs (Klonopin and Effexor) for about 2 1/2 weeks, I cannot wait to see how I'll be feeling a month from now. I thought I'd never get over that dizzy, lightheaded, floating feeling in my head, with the lack of concentration and the agonizing pain in my joints and muscles.

Each day has gotten easier and easier. I had some very hard ones in there, though, but I am so happy I have done this.

The other day, I was teaching a Boot camp class and I had a coat on that I hadn't worn since last fall, I put my hand in my pocket and there was a Klonopin in there. I looked at it and it really made me think. A month ago, if I was in that stressful class situation I would have taken a small bite out of that little pill...instead I threw it away!!!!!

I really am serious about wanting to spread the word about these drugs. I think everything happens for a reason and there's a season for everything. This was the right time for me to stop taking them. I just want others who depend on these medications to be aware and know more of what the doctors are not telling us. Again thank you for helping me get my passion back"

"Today has been the 5th day on the supplements. 10 days with no Klonopin! 12 days with no Effexor! I am feeling a lot of relief from the dizziness/brain zaps and concentration or lack of. Thank God, because that is the worst withdrawal symptom!! I'm sleeping better, very deep and feel very rested. My appetite has decreased YEAH!!! Thank you!!!"

"I read through your site for about one month before trying the products myself. I must say, all of the "Oh, God's" in your testimonials made me wonder if this could really be true. I was told not to really expect a change for 3 to 7 days. After day 1 I had to call TRB Health and tell them what they had here. The "Oh, God" statements I have read now make sense. I was taking an antidepressant and a benzodiazepine and reached the state of no energy, a grinding anxiety during the day, could not sleep at night and more. The Power Barley

Formula and the cherry blew me away. You guys have a spokesperson when you want one. Thank you."

What to Do If You Are Taking Multiple Drugs

If you are taking a benzodiazepine, anti-anxiety or sleep medication along with an antidepressant, anti-psychotic or ADHD medication, deciding which medication to taper off first is important. There are times when a benzodiazepine or sleep medication will have a drug/drug interaction with antidepressants, anti-psychotics and ADHD medications.

Most of the time an antidepressant, anti-psychotic or ADHD medication *will* have a drug-drug interaction with other antidepressant, anti-psychotic or ADHD medication ...but not always. Which drug you wean yourself from first will be largely responsible for your success.

The most common reason these medications have a drug/drug interaction is that they share the same metabolizing route. Two medications trying to go through the same pathway will create a "cumulative" effect of the medications and usually one or both medications will take longer to clear the body.

Imagine 4 linemen from your favorite football team trying to push through the front door of your home, shoulder to shoulder. None of the linemen will back off and let the other pass through first. This is what is happening inside the body.

Occasionally, one medication will *greatly* increase the effect of another medication.

Example: Zoloft and Ambien

Ambien is increased by 43% with concurrent Zoloft usage. You will need to taper off the Ambien *first* or you will go into withdrawal on the Ambien, even though it was not reduced.

First Step in Getting off Multiple Drugs:

Read "The Science Behind The Road Back." The chapter is technical, so take the material to your physician and/ or pharmacist.

Your success will depend on knowing about the drugs you are going to get off, and how (or if) they interact.

If you are taking a benzodiazepine, anti-anxiety or sleep medication with an anti-depressant, anti-psychotic or ADHD medication, *we do need to address the pre-taper differently.*

- Go to the chapter, *Pre-Taper For Antidepressants, Anti-Psychotics and ADHD Medication* and use the pre-taper method titled "If you have anxiety or insomnia." Follow that pre-taper exactly.

Pre-Taper Program if Using an Antidepressant, Anti-Psychotic or ADHD Medication Combination

Use the Pre-Taper for antidepressants, anti-psychotics and ADHD Medication. Use the anxiety and insomnia pre-taper program if that applies.

- The charts in the chapter "The Science Behind The Road Back" must be used to determine which medication to taper off first.

- Once you have fully tapered off a medication, wait 14 days before starting the taper off the next medication. This gives you and your body time to adjust.

To recap: If taking a benzodiazepine along with an antidepressant, anti-psychotic or ADHD medication, use the pre-taper outlined for Antidepressant, Anti-psychotic or ADHD medication if you have anxiety and insomnia.

If you are taking an antidepressant, anti-psychotic or ADHD medication in a combination, use the pre-taper outlined for Antidepressant, Anti-psychotic or ADHD medication and select the pre-taper that fits your individual case.

When reducing any of the medications, use the instructions found for that class of medication. Wait 14 days before reducing the next medication.

Continue taking all supplements as established during the pre-taper.

CHAPTER 16

WHAT CAN BE DONE IF YOU HAVE NEVER TAKEN PSYCHIATRIC MEDICATION

If you are suffering from anxiety, stress that does not seem to end, fatigue or a host of symptoms, you absolutely have an alternative to psychiatric medication.

First: Get a complete physical and have the physician rule out all disease or illness.

There can be life events that were the direct cause of depression, anxiety, stress, fatigue and more. Usually, these feelings go away on their own in a matter of days or weeks without you doing anything other than letting some time pass.

These medications are strong, some are truly addicting, and all of the drugs are life altering. The question is how your life will be altered.

When depression, anxiety, stress, and/or fatigue begin, other factors also play a role in general health. Levels of hormones, adrenals, glucose, cortisol and other functions can become drained, imbalanced or overly stimulated. Psychoactive medications, in part, are designed to regulate all of these functions to some degree, but they ultimately affect these functions by altering other chemicals in the brain and body.

Second: If you are diagnosed with a disease or illness, make sure the diagnosis is from an objective test – not a subjective analysis. As of this writing, all mental disorders are diagnosed with subjective tests.

Later in this chapter you will find possible solutions for symptoms you may be experiencing. One example is using the JNK supplement, Body Calm, Body Calm Supreme and Essential Protein Formula for anxiety symptoms. These supplements do not cure disease or illness. With that in mind, if you feel the anxiety vanish once you begin using these supplements, you must not have had an Anxiety Disorder.

If you were diagnosed with chronic fatigue syndrome, take the JNK supplement, and no longer feel the fatigue, you were misdiagnosed. Misdiagnoses can and do happen.

If a diagnosis of ADHD is presented, then you take Ultimate Omega 3, JNK, vitamin E, and possibly Body Calm and your symptoms subside, you did not have ADHD. Again, these supplements do not cure or prevent disease or illness. If you feel the major positive changes after using these supplements, your body was just lacking those nutrients.

Good-meaning, well-intentioned physicians often feel like they must prescribe psychoactive medication or face the threat of malpractice. One senior partner in a law firm refused to even read this book. Why? His answer was, "If there is a way to taper off psychiatric drugs, with little to no side effects, we would no longer have a case."

If you receive a clean bill of health from your physician, there are suggestions and probable solutions.

Anxiety, Stress, Fatigue, and Depression – Anxiety, stress, fatigue and depression quickly wear the body down. In no time the body begins to feel drained and rundown. One can easily lose track of where the anxiety, stress, fatigue or depression started, and when the body seemed to lump together with your overall feeling.

The goal of The Road Back is to assist you in keeping you separated from the anxiety, stress, fatigue and depression from the body.

As an example, take a finger on your hand.

You can unintentionally hit your finger with a hammer. Your hurt finger will have an effect on you until it heals. You can also decide to hit your finger with a hammer and have an effect on your body.

In either case, if the finger were hit hard enough, you and the injured body part would begin to lump together and you would begin to feel like you were only the body. Or your attention would become so fixed on the body that it would be difficult to distinguish the two. Your entire attention becoming fixated on the hurt finger.

Ask an artist to hit his/her finger with a hammer very hard and to then paint a beautiful picture or create anything not associated with pain. It will not happen. The live, creating part of us, the part that feels emotion – both wanted or unwanted emotion – begins to collapse with the body.

There is not a drug made that can prevent a person from hitting his or her finger with a hammer.

If you have just lost a loved one, or on a lesser scale, just lost your job, there are no supplements or medications that will replace the loss.

The most a psychoactive medication will do is deaden the feelings experienced because of the loss. The most a good supplement will do is assist the body to not succumb to the continued drain put on it because of the feeling of loss.

The Road Back has zero chance of coming into your life and handling the life reason for anxiety, stress, depression or even fatigue. However, we can assist your body to not succumb to the physical stressors being put on it daily from emotional trauma.

Hundreds of clinical trials have shown that people with anxiety; stress, fatigue and depression have low levels of amino acids, vitamins, minerals, antioxidant levels and more. These clinical trials point to the fact that a person will suffer a depletion of these vital nutrients if they are put under enough stress or duress for a period of time.

Our goal here is to point out a few things you can do to help your body maintain general health and well-being while you address the real reason for the problem you are experiencing.

When using the terms anxiety, stress, depression and fatigue, we do not imply a disease or illness associated with these conditions.

If you are trying to choose between two different jobs or changing jobs and feel anxiety and stress, that anxiety or stress is not a disease. After choosing one or the other, the anxiety or stress would vanish. If you just experienced a loss in life, that loss is not a disease. That is part of what eventually happens to each living person. Natural emotions are not diseases or illnesses. You should be considered very sane and normal.

If an emotion continues beyond some arbitrary "they should be over it by now" time period, psychoactive medication comes into play. Neither these drugs nor supplements will help you "realize" or have an "earth shattering realization" about why you have felt that way for such a long time or remove the loss you feel. They will not.

Psychoactive medication may block the emotion, but the emotion will need to be dealt with at some time in the future, unless you just wish to feel "flat-lined" forever. Most people tell us, in hindsight, they would have been better off dealing with the emotion when it happened, instead of putting it off for months or years and then dealing with the emotion on top of the drug withdrawal.

This is why The Road Back suggests using a few supplements. Again, the supplements are not going to solve the problem or underlying condition. They will only help maintain the body's general health and well-being and give you the chance to address the original problem.

We break down symptoms into two areas; anxiety/stress/insomnia, or fatigue. You may feel that you have depression, but even the depression will fit in to one of these two categories.

For Anxiety/Stress/Insomnia: Go to the chapter General Pre-Tapering and Tapering Instructions and read the entire chapter. Then go to the chapter Pre-Taper for Benzodiazepines, Anti-anxiety, Anticonvulsant and Sleep Medication and follow the pre-taper instructions.

Use the Daily Journal and complete the entire pre-taper. This should handle all anxiety, stress and /or insomnia, if present. You can use these supplements as long as you wish; they are not addictive or habit forming.

For Fatigue: Read the entire chapter General Pre-Tapering and Tapering Instructions. Then go to the chapter Pre-Taper for Antidepressants, Antipsychotics and ADHD Medication and follow the pre-taper instructions in the section, *If You Have Fatigue*.

Other Options

There are several excellent products available you can take to get you and your body back in shape again. An example of these products can be found at http://www.theradiantgreens.com. Their Radiant Greens Natural is one of my favorites. Find yourself a good doctor to work with. Maybe a chiropractor or naturopath, who understands nutrition a little more than a medical doctor, is in order.

CHAPTER 17

THE SCIENCE BEHIND
THE ROAD BACK

INTRODUCTION

The Road Back Program and the Development of the Program:

1. There are basic common denominators of psychotropic drug side effects.

2. How our individual DNA affects drug metabolism.

3. The effect of psychotropic medication within the Hypothalamus-Pituitary-Adrenal Axis and immune system.

4. Utilizing DNA clinical trials, test subject trials and psychotropic drug clinical trials to formulate specific nutritional products to eliminate, reduce or avert withdrawal side effects, while not creating drug/supplement interactions.

This research and development complexity has been transformed into an easy to understand, systematic program, which allows an individual to taper off their medication while alleviating a vast percentage of the debilitating side effects of withdrawal.

The sequence of this program and the application of each step is the key to success. Your patient will not begin to reduce a medication until the pre-taper is complete. The pre-taper is a 7-day process.

Statements of fact: All psychoactive medications metabolize through specific pathways. *All* psychoactive medications alter the Hypothalamus Pituitary-Adrenal Axis to some degree. To some extent, you can predict the duration before drug-adverse reactions begin with most psychoactive drugs; if the patient's P450 (CYP) enzymes have been screened.

A poor metabolizer as well as an extensive metabolizer will eventually reach the same saturation point; the poor metabolizer much faster, of course.

If one were to look at the basic structure of the human body, the chemical structure of psychiatric drugs, and include how psychiatric drugs are metabolized, how foods, vitamins, minerals, DNA, amino acids, hormones, glands, proteins, fatty acids and enzymes work, in relation to psychiatric drugs, you have The Road Back Science.

Drug targets for most disorders will be the purinergic system, the dynorphin opioid neuropeptide system, the cholinergic system (muscarinic and nicotinic systems), the melatonin and serotonin system, and the HPA. One reason the supplements were selected to be used in this program, is their natural action of helping to balance the same drug targets.

DNA and Prediction of Drug Adverse Reactions

The following charts detail the P450 enzymes used to metabolize the most common antidepressants, anti-psychotics, benzodiazepines and ADHD stimulant medications. An X in the row denotes that the medication utilizes that specific pathway. Below each chart, you will find other routes of metabolism if applicable.

These medications *inhibit* metabolism via listed CYP pathways.

Drug	P450 Enzyme Pathway				
Antidepressants	1A2	2C19	2C9	2D6	3A
Anafranil	X	X		X	X
Celexa		X		X	
Cymbalta	X			X	
* Elavil	X	X		X	
Effexor				X	X
Lexapro		X		X	
* Luvox	X	X	X	X	X
Pamelor				X	X
* Paxil	X	X	X	X	
* Prozac	X	X	X	X	X
Remeron	X			X	X
Sarafem	X	X	X	X	X
Strattera		X		X	
* Tofranil	X	X		X	X
Trazodone				X	X
* Wellbutrin	X		X	X	X
* Zoloft	X	X	X	X	X

These marked medications (*) will also use other routes for metabolism:

Elavil – UGT1A4, UGT1A3, P-gp

Luvox – 2B6, P-gp, intestinal 3A

Paxil – 2B6, P-gp

Prozac – 2B6, P-gp

Tofranil – UGT1A4, UGT1A3, P-gp

Wellbutrin – 2E1, 2A6, 2B6

Zoloft – UGT2B7, UGT1A4, P-gp, 2B6

Drug	P450 Enzyme Pathway				
Anti-psychotics	1A2	2C19	2C9	2D6	3A
Abilify				X	X
* Clozaril	X	X	X	X	X
* Geodon	X				X
* Haldol	X			X	
* Risperdal				X	X
* Seroquel					X
* Zyprexa	X			X	
Other					
Cogentin				X	
* Lithium					

These marked medications (*) will also use other routes for metabolism:

Clozaril – FMO, UGT1A4, UGT1A3

Geodon – Aldehyde oxidase substrate

Haldol – Glucuronidation, P-gp

Risperdal – P-gp, renal extraction

Seroquel – Glucuronidation, P-gp, intestinal 3A, epoxide by quetiapine

Zyprexa – Glucuronidation, FMO, UGT1A4.

Drug	P450 Enzyme Pathway				
Benzodiazepine Anti-anxiety Sleep Medication	1A2	2C19	2C9	2D6	3A
Ambien	X		X		X
Ativan	UGT2B7				
* BuSpar				X	X
* Depakote	X	X	X		X
Klonopin					X
Librium					X
* Valium		X			X
* Xanax		X			X

These marked medications (*) will also use other routes for metabolism:

BuSpar – Intestinal 3A

Depakote – UGT2B7, UGT1A6, UGT1A9, UGT2B15, UGT1A4, UGT1A3

Valium – 2B6, UGT2B7, intestinal 3A

Xanax – Hepatic 3A.

Drug	P450 Enzyme Pathway				
Stimulants	1A2	2C19	2C9	2D6	3A
Adderall				X	
* Concerta				X	
Dextrostat				X	
* Ritalin				X	

These marked medications (*) will also use other routes for metabolism:

Concerta – Glucuronidation.

Ritalin – Glucuronidation.

How to Use Charts to
Decide Sequence of Medication Reduction

If you have two or more medications sharing the same CYP pathway to metabolize, reduce the medication that uses the fewest pathways first.

Example: Ambien used concurrently with Luvox, Paxil, Prozac, Wellbutrin or Zoloft. Reduce the Ambien first.

If you were to reduce any of the antidepressants listed first, the Ambien would be reduced and the patient would experience Ambien withdrawal without the current Ambien dosage being reduced. Ambien would be reduced by as much as 43% if the antidepressant were reduced first. (See Ambien product insert.)

If taking two antidepressants concurrently, or taking an antidepressant and an antipsychotic, selecting which one to reduce first would also follow the format outlined earlier in this section. The drug using fewer *common* CYP pathways should be reduced first.

If taking two antidepressants or one antidepressant and one antipsychotic, and the CYP pathways match, evaluate the current side effects, when each side effect started, when each medication was introduced, and determine from those side effects which taper schedule to follow.

From time to time, a person will also be taking a drug as an inducer of the CYP pathways.

Determine if this "inducer" was prescribed to help offset the inhibitor drug's effect or is the *inducer* drug prescribed for other health reasons not related.

You will generally find that those who are also taking the *inducer* medication will be suffering from a wide variety of adverse side effects. When reducing any medication attached to the same pathway as an inducer medication, reduce the normal taper speed by one-half for at least the first 2 months.

You may need to alternate reduction of the inducer drug and the inhibitor drug every other reduction in order to maintain a balance.

Other medications must be closely evaluated. Lipitor, as an example, is an inhibitor of the CYP 2C19, 2D6, and 3A, along with inhibiting the UGT1A3, UGT1A1, P-gp, and intestinal 3A.

Use drug product insert to determine metabolism route or the Physicians' Desk Reference.

Example 1: If taking multiple medications and each medication uses the same metabolic route, each of the medications is competing for clearance. If one medication is reduced, the other medications will also be reduced or clear the body faster.

Decide which medication to taper off first based on:

- CYP charts

- full evaluation of side effects

- when side effects started with which medication.

If patient has used Lexapro for two years and used Risperdal for 2 months and side effects increased dramatically once Risperdal was introduced, taper the Risperdal first.

Example 2: If multiple medications are being taken and all medications can metabolize through several routes, the impact will be lessened, and selecting which medication to taper first would not be pathway dependant.

- Avoid all *supplements* that compete with the same pathways, and eliminate as much as possible all foods that compete with the medication by inducing or inhibiting the metabolism routes of the medications.

Supplements, Herbs and Foods

Supplements, herbs or certain foods can have a direct impact on the success of the taper.

Datum: If a person smokes or drinks coffee before starting the pre-taper, do not suggest they quit. Cigarette smoke *induces* the CYP1A2, 2E1, 3A and UGT2B7. Nicotine inhibits UGT1A1, UGT1A4, UGT2A6, and UGT1A9. If taking Depakote and starting or stopping smoking, the impact on the medication will be dramatic

Coffee or caffeine inhibits the CYP1A2, 2E1 and the 3A. A high percentage of these medications metabolize through these pathways and caffeine usage will dramatically increase the medication, or if the person were to quit drinking caffeine, they would begin to go into withdrawal to some degree because the pathways will begin to metabolize the medication faster.

The times a person takes medication and when they drink two cups of coffee can have an impact as well. If the person drinks two cups of coffee every morning about one hour after their medication, and they change the time of the morning they drink the coffee, expect a slight to above average side effect from the medication.

Green tea, with its current popularity is the most problematic at this time. I am not saying green tea is not beneficial. I am saying there is a time and place for supplements, herbs and some specific foods once a person is off all medication for 45 days.

The person's current daily routine should not be changed. If they were on a poor diet before starting this program, do not change their diet drastically. If they did not exercise before starting this program, do not advise them to do more than a casual walk.

Once off all medication for 45 days, a healthy diet can be implemented, an exercise program that matches their current physical condition can be started, the patient can stop smoking, etc.

DNA Drug Reaction Testing and Taper Prediction

For the past several years, DNA drug reaction testing has been available to determine the patient's ability to metabolize medication through the CYP450 enzymes.

I have conducted over 200 drug reaction tests with the objective of determining how well drug-adverse reactions could be predicted, and if there were clinical use of this DNA data for tapering.

Prediction of a drug-adverse reaction: The individuals who were slow or poor metabolizers or hyper metabolizers experienced drug-adverse reactions faster than normal or intermediate metabolizers.

However, the normal or intermediate metabolizers still experienced adverse drug reactions, but after longer usage of the medication. *The metabolism type of the individual was not indicative of the severity of adverse reactions or duration.* Once the drug had saturated the CYP enzyme used for metabolism, all the individuals experienced the same side effect profile regardless of their metabolism speed noted from the DNA drug reaction test.

The test results from the DNA drug-reaction test did not lead to a worthwhile taper guide. It was postulated; if you were to induce the enzymes or inhibit an enzyme to match a specific test result and medication, you would be better able to adjust the metabolism and avoid withdrawal, or predict the withdrawal sequence. Again, this did not assist in tapering or eliminating withdrawal side effects in the slightest. This seems to parallel the results using an *inducer* drug to counteract the inhibition of the main drug.

If a DNA drug-reaction test has any use to a physician, it would be for predicting the dosage of the medication Coumadin. The initial prescription could be limited to a narrow band, and the correct therapeutic dosage would be found in a few weeks, instead of several months.

Nutritional DNA Test

Nutritional DNA testing provided this program substantial information to work with. I tested the ability of over 100 subjects to metabolize B vitamins, folate, calcium, Omega 3, phase II liver detox genes, and an assortment of other genetic differences that ultimately determine overall health and physical well being.

The Road Back Program and all suggested nutritionals used for medication tapering address the most common genetic variations of the population at large. Though DNA science is not precise at this date, enough evidence is available to formulate part of a program to address the highest percentage of the population.

Hypothalamus-Pituitary-Adrenal Axis (HPA)

Psychoactive medications play havoc with the HPA. While benzodiazepines usually help with anxiety for a certain time period, the feedback loop sending incorrect data will eventually cause cortisol levels to increase, and the result will be increased anxiety in the morning and mid-afternoon. Insomnia will usually follow the cortisol level increase. Other psychoactive medications have their own unique side effect profile and ultimate effect upon the HPA.

First year medical school textbooks describe hypothalamus as: "Hypothalamus is homeostasis or maintaining the body's status quo." As an example, blood pressure, body temperature, fluid, the electrolyte balance and body weight are held in a precise value labeled the "set-point." The body's set-point may change over time, but from day to day, the set-point will remain nearly fixed. With the HPA receiving continual input about the state of the body and the ability of the HPA to initiate changes, as anything might sporadically fall out of balance, it is vital for the HPA to have at hand all necessary nutrients to assist with the compensation.

When the HPA is out of balance, you will have a problem with insulin, stress, anxiety, weight gain, thyroid problems, fatigue, unbalanced sexual hormones and countless other body difficulties.

The hormone, ACTH, will eventually become out of balance, as will the other hormones and adrenals.

Psychoactive medication directly alters specific areas within the HPA. Examine any patient using psychoactive medication for more than three months and you will probably find a problem with hormones, thyroid, adrenals, cortisol and immune system or other areas within the HPA.

However, it will be equally important to move beyond the normal view of the HPA. Psychoactive medication side effects are quite varied and diverse. This is not to rehash data from medical school, but to tie in the knowledge gained in the educational process with psychoactive medication.

Some fibers from the optic nerve go directly to a small nucleus within the hypothalamus (suprachiasmatic nucleus). This nucleus regulates circadian rhythms, and couples the rhythms to the light/dark cycles.

The nucleus of the solitary tract will collect sensory data from the vagus and relay the data to the hypothalamus. This data will include blood pressure and gut enlargement.

The reticular formation receives a vast supply of inputs from the spinal cord and relays that data to the hypothalamus. Part of that data will be skin temperature.

Nuclei, circumventricular organs, are unique in their own right as they lack a blood-brain barrier. They monitor substances in the blood and have the ability to monitor substances normally shielded by the neural tissue. Here you will find regulation of fluid and electrolyte balance, by controlling thirst, sodium excretion, blood volume regulation and vasopressin secretion. Include in this the area postrema, and you have the detection of blood toxins and the vomit-inducing center. The OVLT and area postrema project to the hypothalamus.

The limbic and olfactory systems project to the hypothalamus. Psychoactive medication side effects, such as eating problems and reproduction difficulty, will probably be traced to this area.

Ionic balance and temperature will be subject to the hypothalamus via the receptors, thermoreceptor and osmorecepter.

When the hypothalamus is aware of a problem, it will assert repair mechanisms. Neural signals to the autonomic system will attempt to regulate heart rate, vasoconstriction, digestion, sweating etc, and the endocrine signals to and or through the pituitary.

The pituitary side effects will include one or all six hormones, to include ACTH and the thyroid-stimulating hormone (TSH).

The repair output attempt, and the psychoactive medication side effect profile, seem to run near a 50 percent occurrence. Furthermore, you can directly trace psychoactive medication side effects to the autonomic nervous system in both the sympathetic and parasympathetic systems.

The hypothalamus can alter blood pressure; control every endocrine gland in the body, body temperature, adrenal levels via ACTH, and metabolism.

The repetition of HPA information in this chapter has been intentional. Do not be surprised to find a male patient with extremely high estrogen levels, a female with high testosterone or any other problem that can be associated within the HPA.

Taper the medication first, wait 45 days after the last dosage of the medication, reevaluate the patient, and then gradually bring all parts of the HPA back into balance. The nutritionals used with The Road Back Program were developed to help the body overcome this imbalance *gradually*. Gradually is italicized because this is where most problems occur with psychoactive drug-taper programs. Either they do not address the HPA or the program is really a detoxification or heavy metal chelating program.

The Road Back Program utilizes specific nutritionals to address the drug side effects and to begin the process of balancing the HPA. Specifics on each nutritional, what each nutritional is addressing within the HPA or the body in relation to psychoactive medications, can be found in The Road Back Program patent when published by the U.S. Patent Office.

Immune System

The immune system and the HPA are in constant communication and actions within one system will induce response in the other. The supplements used in this program are designed to also influence the immune response.

Reducing oxidative stress has been shown to balance Interleukin-2 (IL-2) as well as Interleukin-6. If you were to test your bipolar patients IL-2 levels, you will find they will be too high during the manic phase and IL-6 levels will have shot up high during the depressive phase. A schizophrenic will have either too high or too low IL-2 levels and will usually exhibit high IL-6 levels constantly.

The JNK supplement will reduce oxidative stress and lower IL-2 levels as well as IL-6 levels.

Titrating Medication

The Road Back has tried titrating medication gradually without the use of nutritionals with limited success. About 50% of the people could taper off their medication without using these nutritionals but they still suffered extreme withdrawal side effects.

Using a gradual titration combined with a basic detoxification approach had lower than 50% success.

The normal supplements used to remove heavy metal or for a liver detox produced undesirable results.

A gradual titration with the use of the suggested nutritionals gives the standard successful results.

The Key to a Successful Taper
With The Road Back Program

Following the pre-taper exactly as described is critical. The pre-taper is the make or break point for *every* successful taper.

Most problems occur when:

- The pre-taper is done too quickly.

- Patient does not stop increasing a nutritional once a positive change occurs.

- Patient changes the time of day they take medication.

- Patient changes the time of day they take nutritionals.

- Medication is reduced too quickly.

- A new medication is prescribed in addition to existing medication.

- Patient is switched to a new medication.

- Doctor has patient use additional supplements or vitamins not in this program.
- Patient begins taking other supplements.
- Patient makes a major change to their daily routine.
- Patient skips days of taking medication.

Titrating Psychoactive Medication:

Have the patient compound his/her medication whenever possible. An exact reduction of the medication each week provides prediction, no guessing, and the highest chance of success.

In the early days of psychoactive drugs, psychiatry did not titrate psychoactive drugs up slowly on patients and the results were catastrophic. Many drugs, other than psychoactive drugs, must be titrated up as well as down before discontinuing.

There seems to be a medical community consensus that psychoactive drugs can be reduced quickly, or patients can abruptly be taken off one psychoactive drug and prescribed another psychoactive drug without an adverse consequence. This is not the case. Even switching a patient from a tablet form of a psychoactive drug to the liquid form of the same psychoactive drug can cause extreme adverse drug reactions.

Dr. Donald E. McAlpine, psychiatrists at the Mayo Clinic states: *"It's important to taper off slowly, extending the taper over several weeks under your physician's direction. When you stop too quickly, you may experience so-called discontinuation symptoms, which can masquerade as relapse."*

The discontinuation process and side effects therein can be confusing to both the patient and physician. Which side effect is coming from the medication, or is it a return of the original symptom?

With a full pre-taper completed before reducing the medication, rest assured the side effect starting during the taper is due to one of the following:

- **The patient changed something.**

- **The reduction of the medication is too large.**

A change made by the patient can be the most difficult to find. It might be something the patient does not feel is a change.

Years ago, I had a person nearly halfway off Paxil. This person experienced no withdrawal side effects tapering the Paxil to that point. When trying to taper off Paxil in the past, the individual had extreme withdrawal side effects after the first reduction attempt and would then need to return to a full dosage.

With no valid explanation, this person began to suffer withdrawal side effect symptoms similar to those earlier. Two weeks passed and I could not find anything the person had changed. Finally, it was mentioned to me by the individual he or she had started an all protein diet, began the diet 3 days before the side effects started.

For this person doing this diet was not a change. He or she would go on this all-protein diet every six months. I give you this example to point out that the change a patient makes may not be so obvious. You may need to dig.

If a patient is keeping a complete Daily Journal these changes can be spotted more quickly and trouble tapering can be avoided.

Use the Suggested Supplements

If you want the standard results with The Road Back Program, use the exact supplements suggested. TRB Health, www.trbhealth.com, (866) 810-3809, has manufactured these supplements to meet our specific requirements for this program.

Why Are These Supplements Used? Here are a few examples.

Body Calm

One of the most common complaints of people trying to come off psychoactive medication is daytime anxiety and the inability to achieve normal sleep at night. Sleep is an integral part of life, helps to stabilize mood, foster clear thinking and assist with reaction time. Sleep gives the body a chance to rebuild. Without plenty of restful sleep, daily functioning can be miserable for the patient.

Body Calm is made from Montmorency cherries and is freeze dried and encapsulated in a veggie capsule.

The Montmorency cherry is a Cox-2 inhibitor. Chronic stress precipitates many neuropsychiatric disorders and alters the various oxidative stress parameters in the brain. Cyclooxygenase (COX) plays an important role in pathogenesis of various neurodegenerative disorders including stroke and seizures.

Behavioral analysis reveals a hyperlocomotor activity and increased anxiety response. Subchronic stress will decrease the percentage of retention of memory and also cause hyperalgesia. Biochemical analysis revealed that chronic immobilization stress significantly increases lipid peroxidation and nitrite levels and will decrease the reduced glutathione and adrenal ascorbic acid levels. Chronic treatment with a Cox inhibitor will significantly attenuate the immobilization stress-induced behavioral and biochemical alterations.

Different from most prescribed medication for anxiety or insomnia, Body Calm does not knock the patient out or sedate. Taken during the day, Body Calm should help relieve anxiety without making the patient tired, foggy or having a feeling of not being alert. Body Calm taken at night, about an hour before bed, will help the patient fall asleep naturally. Upon waking in the morning, the patient will not feel groggy.

Body Calm Supreme

Body Calm Supreme combines 50 mg Body Calm and 200 mg of Passion Flower.

Passion Flower has been shown in several clinical trials during the last decade to handle such things as generalized anxiety, insomnia, and hypertension, withdrawal off benzodiazepines, withdrawal off opiates, narcotics, alcohol and several other addictive substances. Every clinical trial was successful. The same type of Passion Flower used in the clinical trials has been used to formulate Body Calm Supreme.

JNK

The JNK gene becomes over activated with antidepressant usage or when a patient has constant stress, anxiety, panic attacks, heavy metal poisoning, eats fast foods, frozen foods with preservatives, receives X-Ray or U.V. exposure and more. Stopping the over expression of the JNK gene is probably the most vital part of this program.

Reduce the expression of the JNK gene for 30-days and re-evaluate the patient's health and mental outlook. For more information go to www.pubmed.gov and research JNK with any condition.

GLOSSARY

B.I.D.: Twice a day

ACTH: A hormone produced by the pituitary gland that stimulates the secretion of cortisone and other hormones by the adrenal gland. ACTH is also called adrenocorticotropin, corticotropin.

ADHD: Abbreviation for Attention Deficit Hyperactivity Disorder.

ADHD Medication: Medication prescribed for Attention Deficit Hyperactivity Disorder. Common medications are Ritalin, Concerta, Adderall and Strattera.

ADRENAL: The adrenal glands (also known as suprarenal glands) are the triangle-shaped endocrine glands that sit on top of the kidneys; their name indicates that position (*ad-*, "near" or "at" + *-renes*, "kidneys"). They are chiefly responsible for regulating the stress response through a chemical reaction. Adrenaline is a "fight or flight" hormone and plays a central role in short-term stress reaction and is released from the adrenal glands when danger threatens or in an emergency. The adrenal gland also produces Cortisol, a vital hormone often referred to as the "stress hormone" since it is involved in the response to stress. It increases blood pressure, blood sugar levels and can suppress the efficiency of the immune system.

AGITATION: Excitement or emotional disturbance.

ALDEHYDE OXIDASE SUBSTRATE: An enzyme pathway the body uses to metabolize substances.

ALKALINE: Something that is alkaline contains an alkali or has a pH value of more than 7. Your body needs a balance between acid and alkali for good health. When pH levels are too low, it means acid is too high in the body. Human bodies are alkaline by design and acid by function. Maintaining proper alkalinity is essential for life, health, and vitality. Simply put, an imbalance of alkalinity creates a condition favorable to the growth of bacteria, yeast and other unwanted organisms. Leading biochemists and medical physiologists have recognized pH (or the acid-alkaline balance) as a key aspect of a balanced and healthy body.

AMINO ACID: Any of a large group of chemical compounds that join together in various ways to form different proteins necessary for life.

AMINE: A chemical compound containing nitrogen, derived from ammonia. The word "amine" derives from "ammonia." Nitrogen is a biologically important colorless, odorless, tasteless gas. It makes up nearly four fifths of the air around the earth, and is found in all living things. Nitrogen, a constituent of protein, is present in all living cells.

ANTIOXIDANT: Any substance that reduces oxidative damage (damage due to oxygen) such as that caused by free radicals. Here's how oxidation works: As oxygen interacts with cells of any type – an apple slice turning brown, or in your body, the cells lining your lungs or in a cut on your skin – oxidation occurs. This produces some type of change in those cells. They may die, such as with rotting fruit. In the case of cut skin, dead cells are replaced in time by fresh, new cells, resulting in a healed cut. Oxidation reaction can produce free radicals, which start chain reactions that damage cells. Free radicals are highly reactive chemicals that attack molecules by capturing electrons and thus modifying chemical structures. Antioxidants terminate these chain reactions by removing free radicals, and inhibit other oxidation reactions by being oxidized themselves. Well-known antioxidants include a number of enzymes and other substances such as vitamin C, vitamin E and beta carotene (which converts to vitamin A) that are capable of counteracting the damaging effects of oxidation.

Free radicals are atoms or molecules with unpaired electrons. These unpaired electrons are usually highly reactive, so radicals are likely to take part in chemical reactions. When free radicals are on the attack, they don't just kill cells to acquire their missing electron. The problem is that free radicals often injure the cell, damaging the DNA, creating the seed for disease. Free radicals trigger a damaging chain reaction. Free radicals are dangerous because they don't damage just one molecule. One free radical can set off a whole chain reaction. When a free radical oxidizes a fatty acid, it changes that fatty acid into a free radical, which then damages another fatty acid. It's a very rapid chain reaction.

ASSIMILATE: To take something in and make it part of oneself; absorb.

AUDIOGENIC SEIZURES: Seizures caused by loud sounds and noises.

AUTONOMIC NERVOUS SYSTEM: That part of the nervous system specifically concerned with the involuntary, seemingly automatic, activities of organs, blood vessels, glands and a variety of other tissues in the body. The autonomic nervous system breaks down into two subordinate systems that work in conjunction with one another:

the craniosacral and thoracolumbar. See Craniosacral and Thoraco-lumbar in this glossary.

BASKET CASE: Someone not doing well emotionally, very nervous and upset.

BASAL METABOLIC RATE: The rate at which the body uses energy when at rest.

BENZODIAZEPINE PROTRACTED WITHDRAWAL: With-drawal effects from a benzodiazepine that have gone on longer than is normal.

BIOCHEMISTRY: The science dealing with the chemistry of plant and animal life.

BLOOD BRAIN BARRIER (BBB)

A mechanism that controls the passage of substances from the blood into the cerebrospinal fluid (a clear, colorless fluid that bathes the entire surface of the central nervous system and cushions the brain and spinal cord against concussion or violent changes of position) and thus into the brain and spinal cord.

The blood-brain barrier (BBB) lets essential metabolites, such as oxygen and glucose, pass from the blood to the brain and central nervous system (CNS) but blocks most molecules that are more massive. This means that everything from hormones and neuro-transmitters to viruses and bacteria are refused access to the brain by the BBB.

Key functions of the BBB are:

- Protecting the brain from "foreign substances" (such as virus-es and bacteria) in the blood that could injure the brain.

- Shielding the brain from hormones and neurotransmitters in the rest of the body.

- Maintaining a constant environment (homeostasis) for the brain.

BRAIN ZAPS: "Brain zaps" are a withdrawal symptom experienced during discontinuation (or reduction of dose) of SSRI and SNRI (see definitions of SSRI, SNRI in this glossary) antidepressant drugs. They may also be experienced while the person is actually taking the prescribed medication, and can continue for years after withdrawal from the medication.

The experience is hard to explain if never experienced, but brain zaps basically feel like a sudden "jolt" or an electric shock, followed by a few minutes of light-headedness and disorientation. Physiologically, a "brain zap" is a wave-like electrical pulse that quickly travels across the surface of the brain. Brain zaps occur when withdrawing from SSRI and SNRI antidepressants that have an extremely short elimination half-life; that is, they are more quickly metabolized by the liver and leave the general circulation faster than longer half-life antidepressants. This attribute of abruptness leaves the brain a relatively short time to adapt to a major neuron chemical change when the medication is stopped, and the symptoms may be caused by the brain's attempt to readjust.

Carbohydrate: All carbohydrates are made from sugars. There are a number of different types of sugars but in the body all carbohydrate metabolism converts sugar to glucose, our body's preferred energy source. Glucose is the main sugar present in many foods but some contain different sugars, such as fructose in fruit, lactose in milk, as well as others. Most sugars are digested and absorbed and converted to glucose, some cannot be digested. We call this fiber.

Complex Carbohydrate: What are complex carbohydrates?

Complex carbohydrates or starch are simply sugars bonded together to form a chain. The fiber content causes digestive enzymes to work much harder to access the bonds to break the chain into individual sugars for absorption through the intestines.

For this reason digestion of complex carbohydrates takes longer. The slow absorption of sugars provides us with a steady supply of energy and limits the amount of sugar converted into fat and stored. Some examples of complex carbohydrates are vegetables, whole grain breads, whole grain cereals and legumes.

Simple Carbohydrate: Simple carbohydrates are digested quickly. Many simple carbohydrates contain refined sugars and few essential vitamins and minerals. Examples include fruit juice, milk, honey, white bread, white rice, molasses and sugar.

CATCH 22: An impossible situation because you cannot do one thing until you do another thing, but you cannot do the second thing until you do the first thing.

CELLULAR SUPPORT: Anything that helps and supports the cells at a cellular level.

CHANGE: To make or become different in some way.

CHEMISTRY: The chemistry of an organism are the chemical substances that make it up and the chemical reactions that go on inside it.

CHLOROPHYLL: The green coloring matter in plants; sunlight causes it to change carbon dioxide and water into carbohydrates that are the food of the plant.

CIRCADIAN RYHTHMS: Pertaining to a period of about 24 hours. Applied especially to the rhythmic repetition of certain phenomena in living organisms at about the same time each day. *Circadian rhythms* are regular changes in mental and physical characteristics that occur in the course of a day (*circadian* is Latin for "around a day"). Most circadian rhythms are controlled by the body's biological "clock." Disruption to rhythms usually causes a negative effect. Most travelers have experienced the condition known as jet lag, with its associated symptoms of fatigue, disorientation and insomnia. The rhythm is linked to the light-dark cycle. Light and dark cycles being daytime and night time and how they affect the body.

CIRCUMVENTRICULAR ORGAN: The circumventricular organs are regions of the brain where the blood barrier is weak. These regions allow substances to cross into brain tissue more freely and thereby allow the brain to monitor the makeup of the blood. See also Blood Brain Barrier for more information.

COGENTIN: A drug – Benztropine mesylate: benzatropine mesilate (marketed as Cogentin). It is used in patients to reduce the side effects of antipsychotic treatment.

COLD TURKEY: To stop taking drugs or alcohol without any gradient; stopping quickly or abruptly.

COMPOUND: A substance made up of two or more elements.

COMPOUNDING PHARMACY: Pharmacy is regarded as the science of compounding and dispensing medication; also an establishment used for such purposes. Modern pharmaceutical practice includes the dispensing, identification, selection, and analysis of drugs. Compounding pharmacies are on the rise and physicians, medical institutions and patients are realizing more than ever the importance of tailoring an individual's medications to specifically meet their needs. A majority of the pharmacists that are going back to compounding are doing so for the love of the science and interest in the patient's well being. The role of a problem solver opens the door to creativity and genius.

CONJUGATED LINOLEIC ACID (CLA): An unsaturated omega-6 fatty acid.

CONSTANT LEVEL: To maintain a level of a supplement in the body to a degree where it never drops below a certain point.

CONTRA: In opposition to; against.

CONTRASURVIVAL: Opposition to or against survival.

CORTISOL: A hormone produced in the adrenal glands. A vital hormone often referred to as the "stress hormone" as it is involved in the response to stress. It increases blood pressure, blood sugar levels and can reduce the efficiency of the immune system. The synthetic form of cortisol is referred to as hydrocortisone.

CORTISOL LEVELS: Cortisol levels can be too high or too low, each causing problems within the body and hormone balance.

COUMADIN: Coumadin is an anticoagulant (blood thinner) which reduces the formation of blood clots by blocking the synthesis of certain clotting factors. Without these clotting factors, blood clots cannot form. Coumadin is used to prevent heart attacks, strokes, and blood clots in veins and arteries.

CRANIOSACRAL: Pertaining to the craniosacral system. That part of the nervous system concerned mainly with the body's everyday function of excreting waste products. Most active during sleep, slows the heart rate and stimulates the organs of the digestive system because the nerves of this system originate from two regions – the cranial (cranial, meaning of the skull) and sacral (sacral, meaning in the area of the sacrum, a bone at the lower end of the spine forming the back portion of the pelvis).

CUMULATIVE EFFECT: A series of events having a cumulative effect, each event increases the effect.

CYP PATHWAY: An enzyme pathway the body uses to metabolize substances such as drugs. For more information see intermediate metabolizer.

CYP 2D6: An enzyme pathway the body uses to metabolize substances such as drugs.

CYP 2C19: An enzyme pathway the body uses to metabolize substances such as drugs.

CYP 3A: An enzyme pathway the body uses to metabolize substances such as drugs.

DAILY JOURNAL: An account on which you write your daily activities.

DETOXIFICATION: The act of removing all the poisonous or harmful substances from something.

DEVIATION: Doing something that is different from what people consider normal or acceptable.

DISCONTINUATION SYMPTOMS: The side effects or reactions people get when stopping a drug.

DHA: (Docosahexanoic) Docosahexaenoic acid commonly known as **DHA**; it is an omega-3 essential fatty acid. Essential fatty acids, or EFAs, are fatty acids that cannot be constructed within an organism from other components (generally all references are to humans) by any known chemical pathways; and therefore must be obtained from diet. The term refers to those involved in biological processes, and not fatty acids which may just play a role as fuel.

DNA: Deoxyribonucleic acid (DNA) DNA contains the genetic information for the reproduction of life. DNA is a nucleic acid that contains the genetic instructions used in the development and functioning of all known living organisms and some viruses. The main role of DNA molecules is the long-term storage of information. DNA is often compared to a set of blueprints or a recipe, since it contains the instructions needed to construct other components of cells, such as proteins. The DNA segments that carry this genetic information are called genes, but other DNA sequences have structural purposes, or are involved in regulating the use of this genetic information.

DOUBLE-BLIND RANDOMIZED CONTROLLED TRIALS: Double-blind: Term used to describe a study in which both the investigator or the participant are blind to (unaware of) the nature of the treatment the participant is receiving. Double-blind trials are thought to produce objective results, since the expectations of the researcher and the participant about the experimental treatment such as a drug do not affect the outcome.

DRUG/DRUG INTERACTION: The interaction between one drug and another drug and the effect created.

DRUG INSERTS: Material, called package inserts, providing information on the usage and risks of medications – including warnings, side effects, contraindications and interactions with other drugs. The FDA says it is concerned that the old format, plus information overload, mean that some of the information may not be getting through to doctors and consumers, resulting in thousands of "preventable adverse events" every year.

DRUG/SUPPLEMENT INTERACTIONS: The interaction between a drug and a supplement and the effect created.

ELECTROLYTE BALANCE: Electrolyte is a "medical/scientific" term for salts, specifically ions. The term electrolyte means this ion is electrically-charged and moves to either a negative or positive electrode.

Electrolytes are important because they are what your cells (especially nerve, heart, muscle) use to maintain voltages across cell membranes and carry electrical impulses (nerve impulses, muscle contractions) across themselves and to other cells. Your kidneys work to keep the electrolyte concentrations in your blood constant despite changes in your body. For example, when you exercise heavily, you lose electrolytes in your sweat, particularly sodium and potassium. These electrolytes must be replaced to keep body fluids electrolyte concentrations constant.

Electrolyte levels can become too low or too high which can happen when the amount of water in your body changes. Causes include some medicines, vomiting, diarrhea, sweating or kidney problems. Problems most often occur with levels of sodium, potassium or calcium.

ELECTRONICS: The branch of physics that deals with electrons in motion.

EMOTIONAL: Concerned with feelings and emotions.

ENDOCRINE: The system of glands that produce hormones Endocrine glands release hormones (chemical messengers) into the bloodstream to be transported to various organs and tissues throughout the body.

EPA: Eicosapentaenoic acid (EPA) is an omega-3 fatty acid.

ESTROGEN: A female hormone produced primarily in the ovaries. Some estrogens are also produced in smaller amounts by other tissues such as the liver, adrenal glands and the breasts. These secondary sources of estrogen are especially important in postmenopausal women. Estrogen deficiency can lead to osteoporosis (a condition in which bones lose calcium and become more likely to break).

EXACERBATE: If something exacerbates a problem, it makes it worse.

EXTENSIVE METABOLIZER: Approximately half of all Americans have genetic defects that affect how they process drugs. There are four different types of metabolizers. We all fall into one of these categories for the variable pathways in Cytochrome P450 (this Cytochrome is responsible for creating the enzymes that process chemicals of all kinds through our bodies.) The easiest way to understand this is to picture a two lane highway. If you are the first type which is the norm, you would be an EXTENSIVE metabolizer. Both lanes of the highway are open and moving. Medications prescribed in normal doses will be metabolized by your body.

EXTREME: To the greatest degree; very great; excessive. 2. farthest away 3. far from what is usual.

FEEDBACK LOOP: Feedback is both a mechanism, process and signal that is looped back to control a system within itself. This loop is called the feedback loop. A control system usually has input and output to the system; when the output of the system is fed back into the system as part of its input, it is called the "feedback." In a feedback loop, increased amounts of a substance – for example, a hormone – inhibit the release of more of that substance, while decreased amounts of the substance stimulate the release of more of that substance.

FLAT LINED: A flatline is an electrical time sequence measurement that shows no activity and therefore when represented, shows a flat line instead of a moving one. This term almost always refers to either a flatlined electrocardiogram, where the heart shows no electrical activity, or to a flat electroencephalogram, in which the brain shows no electrical activity (brain death). Both of these specific cases are involved in various definitions of death. Some consider one who has flatlined to have been clinically dead, regardless of their eventual resuscitation or lack thereof, whereas others insist that one is alive until the moment of brain death. Term mostly used in the medical industry when a person's pulse has stopped, indicating a flat line on the heart monitor. Flat-lined in this book is used figuratively to mean having no emotion or feeling.

FRAY: fight, battle, or skirmish; a noisy quarrel or brawl.

FREE-RADICAL: Atoms or molecules with unpaired electrons. These unpaired electrons are usually highly reactive, so radicals are likely to take part in chemical reactions. When free radicals are on the attack, they don't just kill cells to acquire their missing molecule. Free radicals often injure the cell, damaging the DNA, which creates the seed for disease. Free radicals trigger a damaging chain reaction. Free radicals are dangerous because they don't just damage one molecule. One free radical can set off a whole chain reaction. When a free radical oxidizes a fatty acid, it changes that fatty acid into a free radical, which then damages another fatty acid. It's a very rapid chain reaction.

FMO: An enzyme pathway the body uses to metabolize substances such as drugs.

GLUCOSE (Glc): A monosaccharide (or simple sugar) also known as grape sugar; an important carbohydrate. The living cell uses it as a source of energy. Glucose is one of the main products of photosynthesis (Photosynthesis is the conversion of light energy into chemical energy by living organisms) and starts cellular respiration (Cellular respiration – the reactions and processes that take place in a cell or across the cell membrane to release energy from nutrients and then release waste products). The name comes from the Greek word *glykys* (γλυκύς), meaning "sweet", plus the suffix "-ose" denoting a sugar.

GLUCARONIC ACID: An acid formed by the oxidation of glucose, found combined with other products of metabolism in the blood and urine.

GLUCURONIDATION: A phase II detoxification pathway occurring in the liver in which glucuronic acid is joined together with toxins. It effectively detoxifies the majority of commonly prescribed drugs. Thus, glucuronidation represents a major means of converting most drugs, steroids and many toxic substances to metabolites that can then be excreted into the urine or bile.

GLUTATHIONE (GSH): A naturally occurring protein that protects every cell, tissue and organ from toxic free radicals and disease. It is a tripeptide of three amino acids - glycine, glutamate (glutamic acid) and cysteine (tripeptide is a peptide consisting of three amino acids). These precursors (precursors are substances from which something else is formed) are necessary for the manufacture of glutathione within the cells. Glutathione has been called the "master antioxidant" and regulates the actions of lesser antioxidants such as vitamin C and vitamin E within the body.

Peptide: A molecule consisting of 2 or more amino acids. Peptides are smaller than proteins, which are also chains of amino acids. Molecules small enough to be synthesized from the constituent amino acids are, by convention, called peptides rather than proteins.

GUT: The stomach or belly.

HALF-LIFE: If you draw a graph of drug levels in the blood, you will see that they rise quickly after a dose is taken, then fall off over time until the next dose. When this blood level drops by 50% that would be half-life.

HAMILTON ANXIETY SCORE: The Hamilton Anxiety Scale (HAS or HAMA) is a 14-item test measuring the severity of anxiety symptoms. It is also sometimes called the Hamilton Anxiety Rating Scale (HARS). The score would be the result of the test with a number value.

HAY FEVER: Allergy caused by the pollen of ragweed, trees, grasses and other plants, characterized by itching, and running eyes and nose and fits of sneezing.

HEAVY METAL CHELATING: Introduction of certain substances into the body so that they will chelate, and then remove, foreign substances such as lead, cadmium, arsenic and other heavy metals. Chelation therapy can also be used to reduce or remove calcium-based plaque from the linings of the blood vessels, easing the flow of blood to vital organs and tissues. *Chelation* is a chemical process by which a larger molecule or group of molecules surround or enclose a mineral atom. One source defines "heavy metal" as common transition metals, such as copper, lead and zinc. These metals are a cause of environmental pollution (heavy-metal pollution) from a number of sources, including lead in petrol, industrial waste, and leaching of metal ions from the soil into lakes and rivers by acid rain.

HEPATIC 3A: Hepatic means having to do with the liver, *see CYP 3A.*

HOMEOSTASIS: The tendency to maintain, or the maintenance of, normal, internal stability in an organism by coordinated responses of the organ systems that automatically readjust for environmental changes.

HORMONES: Essential substances produced by the endocrine glands that regulate bodily functions; a regulatory substance produced in an organism and transported in tissue fluids such as blood to stimulate cells or tissues into action. Hormones are chemicals released by cells that affect cells in other parts of the body. Only a small amount of hormone is required to alter cell metabolism. Also act as chemical messengers that transport a signal from one cell to another.

HPA: The Hypothalamus-Pituitary-Adrenal (HPA) axis is one of the key parts of the human endocrine system. As its name suggests, it comprises three endocrine glands, the hypothalamus, the (anterior) pituitary, and the adrenal gland cortex.

Hypothalamic-Pituitary-Adrenal Axis

What is the HPA axis?

The hypothalamus is the control center for most of body's hormonal systems. Cells in the hypothalamus produce hormone corticotrophin-releasing factor (CRF) in humans in response to most any type of stress – physical or psychological.

The hypothalamus secretes CRF, which in turn binds to specific receptors on pituitary cells, which produce adrenocorticotropin hormone (ACTH). ACTH is then transported to its target the adrenal gland. The adrenal gland then stimulates the production of adrenal hormones which increase the secretion of cortisol.

The release of cortisol initiates a series of metabolic effects aimed at alleviating the harmful effects of stress through negative feedback to both the hypothalamus and the anterior pituitary, which decreases the concentration of ACTH and cortisol in the blood once the state of stress subsides.

HYPER: A prefix meaning over, more than normal, too much.

HYPERAGGRESSION: Too much aggression.

HYPERKINESIAS: An abnormal increase in muscular activity, hyperactivity, especially in children.

HYPER METABOLIZER: Someone that metabolizes too much.

HYPERTHERMIA: Unusually high body temperature.

HYPOTHALAMUS: The hypothalamus links the nervous system to the endocrine system via the pituitary gland. The hypothalamus is located below the thalamus, just above the brain stem. It is also responsible for the motivation of what has been called the "Four F's"(feeding, fighting, fleeing and sexual reproduction (fertility).

The hypothalamus controls body temperature, hunger, thirst, fatigue, anger and circadian cycles.

HYPOTHALAMUS-PITUITARY-ADRENAL AXIS: See HPA

IMMUNE SYSTEM: A complex system that depends on the interaction of many different organs, cells, and proteins. Its chief function is to identify and eliminate foreign substances such as harmful bacteria that have invaded the body. The liver, spleen, thymus, bone marrow and lymphatic system all play vital roles in the proper functioning

INDUCER: An inducer is a molecule that starts gene expression. **Gene expression** is the process by which inheritable information from a gene, such as the DNA sequence, is made into a functional gene product, such as protein.

INFLAMMATORY: Inflammation of the body. Inflammation is a localized physical condition with heat, swelling, redness and usually pain especially as a reaction to injury or infection.

INHIBITOR DRUGS: A drug which restrains or retards physiological, chemical, or enzymatic action.

INSOMNIA: Inability to sleep; abnormal wakefulness.

INSULIN: A protein hormone formed in the pancreas and secreted into the blood, where it regulates carbohydrate (sugar) metabolism.

INTERLEUKIN: Interleukins are a group of cytokines (secreted signaling molecules) that were first seen to be expressed by white blood cells (leukocytes, hence the *-leukin*) as a means of communication (*inter-*). Interleukins are produced by a wide variety of bodily cells. The function of the immune system depends in a large part on *interleukins.*

INTERLEUKIN 6 (IL-6): Made by the body, interleukin-6 (IL-6) is a type of protein that helps regulate the immune system. It can also serve as a liver cell growth factor. IL-6 is needed in the body. However, too much IL-6 will promote inflammation and has been shown to be a direct link to chronic depression.

INTERLEUKIN 2(IL-2): Interleukin-2 is a type of protein found in the immune system that is instrumental to the body's natural response to microbial infection and in discriminating between foreign and self.

INTERMEDIATE METABOLIZER: Of all the clinical factors that alter a person's response to drugs (age, sex, weight, general health and liver function, etc.) genetic factors are the most important. This information becomes crucial when you consider that adverse reactions to prescription drugs are killing about 106,000 Americans each year – roughly three times as many killed by automobiles.

Approximately half of all Americans have genetic defects that affect how they process drugs. There are four different types of metabolizers. We all fall into one of these categories for the variable pathways in Cytochrome P450 (this Cytochrome is responsible for creating the enzymes that process chemicals of all kinds through our bodies).

The easiest way to understand this is to picture a two-lane highway.

If you are the second type, you would be an INTERMEDIATE metabolizer. This means that one lane of that highway is open and moving and the other lane is not, causing you to metabolize the medications more slowly. In this case you will need a lower dosage, and there is a chance of medications building up in your system causing adverse effects. Monitoring medications is especially important if you are in this category.

INTESTINAL 3A: An enzyme pathway the body uses to metabolize substances such as drugs.

INTRACELLULAR: Intra means occurring within; intracellular means occurring within the cell.

IONIC BALANCE: (or electrolyte balance) Balance of fluid in the body fluid compartments; total body water, blood volume, maintained by processes in the body that regulate the intake and excretion of water and electrolytes, particularly sodium and potassium.

ION: an atom or group of atoms having a charge of positive or negative electricity.

IONIC CALCIUM: Ionic means pertaining to ions. Ionic calcium would be calcium that is electrically charged. The type of calcium that fizzes when put it in water. The body breaks down calcium and will turn it ionic through the process of absorption. Using ionic calcium bypasses this action of the body.

IRRITABLE BOWEL SYNDROME (IBS): Irritable bowel syndrome (IBS) is a bowel disorder characterized by mild to severe abdominal pain, discomfort, bloating and alteration of bowel habits. In some cases, the symptoms are relieved by bowel movements.

JOURNAL: A daily record of events.

KRILL: Small, shrimp-like fish that swim in the sea.

LECITHIN: A fatlike substance produced daily by the liver if the diet is adequate. Lecithin is needed by every cell in the body and is a key building block of cell membranes. Without lecithin, cells would harden. Lecithin protects cells from oxidation and largely comprises the protective sheaths surrounding the brain. It is composed mostly of B vitamins, phosphoric acid, choline, linoleic acid and inositol.

LIFE: The quality that distinguishes a vital and functional being from a dead body or inanimate matter.

LIGHT/DARK CYCLES: see Circadian Rhythms.

LIMBIC SYSTEM: The limbic system is a term for a set of brain structures that support a variety of functions including emotion, behavior and long term memory. The structures of the brain described by the limbic system are closely associated with the sense of smell structures. The term "limbic" comes from Latin *limbus*, meaning "border" or "belt."

LYMPH SYSTEM: Part of the immune system with lymph nodes and tissues. The role of tissue fluid is to deliver the groceries to the cells. The role of lymph is to take out the trash that is left behind and dispose of it.

As lymph continues to circulate between the cells it collects waste products that were left behind including dead blood cells, pathogens and cancer cells. This clear fluid also becomes protein-rich as it absorbs dissolved protein from between the cells.

MACROECONOMICS: Macro is added to words that refer to things that are large in size or broad in scope. Macroeconomics means relating to the major, general features of a country's economy such as unemployment and interest rates.

MAJOR CHANGE: A change that is significant.

MAJOR IMPROVEMENTS: An improvement that is significant.

MAJOR POSITIVE CHANGE: A change that is significant and for the better.

MEDICATION INDUCED SIDE EFFECTS: Side effects caused by medication.

MELATONIN: A hormone produced by the pineal gland, intimately involved in regulating the sleeping and waking cycles among other processes. Melatonin supplements are sometimes used by people to handle chronic insomnia. Always see your doctor before taking melatonin, as it is not always recommended for sleep problems.

MEMBRANE: A thin layer of tissue which covers a surface or divides a space or organ.

METABOLIZING ROUTE: An enzyme pathway used to metabolize something in the body.

MINERALS: An inorganic substance required by the body in small quantities.

MUCUS LINING: The moist lining of a body cavity or structure, such as the mouth or nose.

NARCOTICS: Drugs such as opium or heroin which induce sleep and inhibit pain sensation.

NATUROPATH: A health care practitioner that uses diet, herbs and other natural methods and substances to cure illness. The goal is to produce a healthy body state by stimulating innate defenses and without the use of drugs.

NEURAL TISSUE: Neural means pertaining to a nerve or to the nerves. Neural tissue is specialized for the conduction of electrical impulses that convey information or instructions from one region of the body to another. About 98% of neural tissue is concentrated in the brain and spinal cord, the control centers for the nervous system.

NORMAL METABOLIZER: See extensive metabolizer.

NUCLEI: Plural of nucleus

NUCLEUS: The small mass at the center of most living cells.

NUTRIENT: A substance that is needed by the body to maintain life and health.

OLFACTORY SYSTEM: The sensory system used for the sense of smell

OPIATES: A remedy containing or derived from opium; also any drug that induces sleep.

OSMORECEPTER: A specialized sensory nerve ending sensitive to stimulation giving rise to the sensation of odors.

OVLT: The organum vasculosum of the lamina terminalis (OVLT) is one of the circumventricular organs of the brain. Circumventricular organs are so named because they are positioned at distinct sites around the margin of the ventricular system of the brain. The ventricular system is a set of structures in the brain continuous with the central canal of the spinal cord. See Circumventricular organs.

PARASYMPATHETIC SYSTEM: The part of the autonomic nervous system originating in the brain stem and the lower part of the spinal cord that, in general, inhibits or opposes the physiological effects of the sympathetic nervous system, as in tending to stimulate digestive secretions, slow the heart, constrict the pupils and dilate blood vessels. The Sympathetic Nervous System is a branch of the autonomic nervous system. It is always active and becomes more active during times of stress. Its actions during the stress response are the opposite of the parasympathetic system which is to expand pupils, accelerate heart beat, inhibit digestion and relax the bladder. The autonomic nervous system acts as a control system, maintaining balance in the body.

PATHWAY: A particular course of action; *medical;* The sequence of enzymatic steps in the process by which something is metabolized in the body.

P450 (CYP) ENZYMES: An enzyme pathway the body uses to metabolize substances such as drugs.

P-gp: An enzyme pathway the body uses to metabolize substances.

PHASE II LIVER DETOX GENES: To be effective a detox diet must do a few things. First and foremost, a detox diet must increase the phase II of the liver. The liver uses two phases to breakdown chemical toxins.

Phase I: At the end of phase I the liver has accumulated the toxins but they are now in their raw state. This is the stage where your body is the most exposed to toxins. The liver is now holding the toxins in their most toxic state.

Phase II: The liver passes the toxins over to the phase II process. If the phase II process is not functioning properly, the toxins will not be removed and the raw toxins may be dumped back into the body. Phase II is where the toxins are carried out of the body. It is vital during a liver detox that phase II is fully activated. It is also during phase II that glutathione comes into play. Glutathione being activated is every bit as vital during the phase II process of a detox.

There are probably as many viewpoints about how to detox as there are products being sold to handle a detox. However, it does come down to only two actions within the liver, phase I and phase II, the breaking down of toxins and moving them out of the body.

There are 3 genes that regulate the phase II of the liver. The gene names are: GSTM1, GSTT1, and GSTP1. The G stands for Glutathione. At least 50% of the population will have 1 or more of these genes with a variation. The people with a variation in their detox genes will have a more difficult time removing toxins and will need help making glutathione within the liver.

PHOSPHOLIPIDS: Phospholipids are the building blocks of *every cell* in the human body and that includes nerve cells, tissues, blood vessels and skin. Phospholipids protect the body from free-radical attack and toxic injury.

PHYSICAL STRESSORS: Physical Stressors result from internal physical symptoms, such as headaches, stomach problems, etc. and external physical stressors, such as heat, cold, excessive noise, etc.

PLATELETS: A circular oval disk found in the blood which is concerned with coagulation (clotting the blood to stop a wound's bleeding).

POOR METABOLIZER: Approximately half of all Americans have genetic defects that affect how they process these drugs. There are four different types of metabolizers. We all fall into one of these categories for the variable pathways in Cytochrome P450 (this Cytochrome is responsible for creating the enzymes that process chemicals of all kinds through our bodies). The easiest way to understand this is to picture a two lane highway.

If you are the first type which is the norm, you would be an EXTENSIVE metabolizer. Both lanes of the highway are open and moving. Medications prescribed in normal doses will be metabolized by your body.

The third type is a POOR metabolizer. In this case both lanes of the highway would be stopped. There is a possibility that alternate routes can be found, but this type of metabolization is potentially very dangerous, as there is a great chance for the medication to build up in your system making you very sick, or even killing you.

For example, a poor metabolizer of Phenytoin, a common anti-seizure medication would not be able to process the drug and would actually have an increased rather than decreased risk of seizure if prescribed this drug.

POSTREMA: The area postrema is a part of the brain that controls vomiting. The area postrema detects toxins in the blood and acts as a vomit inducing center.

POST TRAUMATIC STRESS DISORDER (PTSD): An anxiety disorder that can develop after exposure to one or more terrifying events in which grave physical harm occurred or was threatened. It is a severe and ongoing emotional reaction to an extreme psychological trauma. The stressor may involve someone's actual death or a threat to the patient's or someone else's life, serious physical injury, or threat to physical and/or psychological integrity, to a degree with which usual psychological defenses cannot cope. In some cases it can also be from profound psychological and emotional trauma, apart from any actual physical harm. Often, however, the two are combined.

PRE-TAPER: Pre means before and taper means to gradually reduce in size or amount. Pre-taper is something you do before a taper.

PROPRIETARY: Owned by a person or company, as under a patent, trademark or copyright.

PROSURVIVAL: Pro means to support, be in favor of; for. Prosurvival means to support or be in favor or survival.

PROTOCOL: Is a course of treatment for someone who is ill or has an addiction.

PROTRACTED: When something has gone on longer than is usual or expected, usually something unpleasant.

PSYCHOACTIVE MEDICATIONS: A psychoactive drug or psychotropic substance is a chemical substance that acts primarily upon the central nervous system where it alters brain function, resulting in temporary changes in perception, mood, consciousness and behavior.

PSYCHOSIS: A psychiatric term for a mental state often described as involving a "loss of contact with reality." People suffering from it are said to be psychotic.

People experiencing psychosis may report hallucinations or delusional beliefs, and may exhibit personality changes and disorganized thinking. This may be accompanied by unusual or bizarre behavior, as well as difficulty with social interaction and impairment in carrying out the activities of daily living.

A wide variety of central nervous system diseases, from both external toxins and from internal physiologic illness, can produce symptoms of psychosis.

PSYCHOTROPIC: Having an altering effect on perception, emotion, or behavior. Used especially of a drug.

PHYSIOLOGY: The scientific study of how human and animal bodies function and how plants function.

PREBIOTICS: Indigestible carbohydrates that stimulate the growth and activity of beneficial bacteria (probiotics) of the intestinal flora.

PROBIOTICS: Your body contains billions of bacteria and other microorganisms. The term "probiotics" refers to dietary supplements or foods that contain beneficial or "good" bacteria similar to those normally found in the body. Although you don't need probiotics to be healthy, these microorganisms may provide some of the same health benefits that the bacteria already existing in your body do – such as assisting with digestion and helping protect against harmful bacteria.

PTSD: See Post Traumatic Stress Disorder.

QUANDARY: State of being uncertain; dilemma.

REACH: 1. To extend out. 2. To touch or to seize 3. To communicate with.

RECEPTORS: Nerve endings in the body which react to changes and stimuli and make your body respond in a particular way.

RELAPSE: To fall back into an earlier condition.

RENAL EXTRACTION: The term "renal" refers to the kidneys. Testing waste coming out of the body to see how much of a drug or substance was left in the body and what is not.

RETICULAR FORMATION: The reticular formation is a part of the brain that is involved in actions such as waking/sleeping cycle and lying down. It is essential for governing some of the basic functions of higher organisms, and is one of the oldest portions of the brain. A network of nerve fibers and cells in parts of the brainstem, important in regulating consciousness or wakefulness.

ROLLED A SEVEN: To get lucky by chance.

SCENARIO: A likely or possible scenario means the way in which a situation may or has developed.

SCORED: "Tablets are scored." Scoring a surface with something sharp means cutting or scratch a line in it.

SELF MEDICATE: Self-medication is the use of drugs to treat a perceived or real malady. Over-the-counter drugs are a form of self medication. The buyer diagnoses his/her own illness and buys a specific drug to treat it. The World Self-Medication Industry (WSMI) defines self-medication as *the treatment of common health problems with medicines especially designed and labeled for use without medical supervision and approved as safe and effective for such use.* A person may also self-medicate by taking more or less than the recommended dose of a drug.

SET-POINT: An arbitrary point for each individual and within each individual's body. The various hormones and endocrine etc. have their own point of reference that is ideal for that body.

7 RATING: A rating on how you are doing kept in your journal on The Road Back Program. A 7-10 rating is a rating that you are doing well. You rate how you feel, your energy, appetite, mood and exercise.

SHORT CHAIN FATTY ACIDS: Fatty acids taken up directly to the portal vein (a large vein that carries blood from the digestive tract to the liver) during digestion of fat. Produced when dietary fiber is fermented in the colon.

SIDE EFFECTS: Problems that occur when treatment goes beyond the desired effect or problems that occur in addition to the desired therapeutic effect.

Example – A hemorrhage from the use of too much anticoagulant (such as heparin) is a side effect caused by treatment going beyond the desired effect.

Example – Common side effects of cancer treatment including fatigue, nausea, vomiting, decreased blood cell counts, hair loss and mouth sores. They occur in addition to the desired therapeutic effect.

Drug manufacturers are required to list all known side effects of their products.

SLEEP MEDICATION: A drug that puts you to sleep.

SLOW METABOLIZER: See poor metabolizer.

SNRI: Serotonin-norepinephrine reuptake inhibitors (SNRIs) are a class of antidepressant used in the treatment of major depression and other mood disorders. Also sometimes used to treat anxiety disorders, obsessive-compulsive disorder, attention deficit hyperactivity disorder (ADHD) and chronic neuropathic pain.

SOLUBLE: Can be dissolved in a liquid.

SSRI: Selective serotonin reuptake inhibitors (SSRIs) are a class of antidepressants used in the treatment of depression, anxiety disorders and some personality disorders. They are also used in treating premature ejaculation problems as well as some cases of insomnia

STAGE 1 DETOXIFICATION: You have completed Stage 1 Detoxification by coming off the medications.

STAGE 2 DETOXIFICATION: The process of removing the remaining toxins from the body. There will be drug toxins remaining in the body as well other toxins picked up by living on planet earth.

STAGE 2 SLEEP: In this stage (the beginning of "true" sleep) the person's electroencephalogram (EEG) will show distinctive wave forms. About 50% of sleep time is stage 2 sleep. Electroencephalography (EEG) is the measurement of electrical activity produced by the brain.

STEADY STATE: A constant level or a level of action that allows a balance between two or more substances.

SUPER FOODS: Highly nutritious supplements considered to have a complete array of all vitamins, minerals and amino acids the human body may need.

SUPRACHIASMATIC NUCLEUS: The suprachiasmatic nucleus (SCN) is a region of the brain (located in the hypothalamus) responsible for controlling from within the body circadian rhythms (see circadian rhythms). The neuronal and hormonal activities it generates regulate many different body functions over a 24-hour period. The suprachiasmatic nucleus of the hypothalamus (SCN) contains a master circadian pacemaker. Biological rhythms are synchronized by light and darkness.

SYMPATHETIC SYSTEM: Sympathetic nervous system is a branch of the autonomic nervous system. Always active, it becomes more active during times of stress. Its actions during the stress response are the opposite of the parasympathetic system which is to expand pupils, accelerate heart beat, inhibit digestion and relax the bladder. The autonomic nervous system acts as a control system, maintaining balance in the body.

SYSTEMATIC: Done according to a fixed plan, in a thorough and efficient way.

SYSTEMIC: Having to do with the body as a whole. Systemic chemicals or drugs are absorbed into the whole of the body rather than being applied to one area.

TAPER: To gradually become reduced in amount, number or size until it is greatly reduced.

TESTOSTERONE: A white crystalline steroid hormone, produced primarily in the testes and responsible for the development and maintenance of male secondary sex characteristics. Also produced synthetically for use in medical treatments.

THERMORECEPTOR: Sensory receptor that responds to heat and cold.

Sensory receptors account for our ability to see, hear, taste and smell, and to sense touch, pain, temperature and body position. They also provide the unconscious ability of the body to detect changes in blood volume, blood pressure, and the levels of salts, gases and nutrients in the blood.

These specialized cells are exquisitely adapted for the detection of particular physical or chemical events outside the cell. They are connected to nerve cells, or are themselves nerve cells.

THORACOLUMBAR: Pertaining to the thoracolumbar system. That part of the nervous system mainly concerned with preparing the body for action particularly during times of stress, excitement or fear. It acts to stimulate such functions as heart rate, sweating and blood flow to the muscles while at the same time decreasing the activity of the digestive system. Called the thoracolumbar system because the nerves of this system originate from two regions of the spine: the thoracic (meaning of the thorax, that area of the body between the neck and the abdomen; chest) and the lumbar (meaning of the lower part of the back below the thorax).

THYROID: A small gland, normally weighing less than one ounce, located in the front of the neck. Made up of two halves, called lobes, that lie along the windpipe (trachea) joined together by a narrow band of thyroid tissue, known as the isthmus.

The thyroid is situated just below the "Adams apple" or larynx. During development (inside the womb) the thyroid gland originates in the back of the tongue, but normally migrates to the front of the neck before birth. Very rarely it fails to migrate properly and is located high in the neck or even in the back of the tongue (lingual thyroid). Also very rarely at other times it may migrate too far and ends up in the chest.

The thyroid gland takes iodine, found in many foods, and converts it into thyroid hormones: thyroxine (T4) and triiodothyronine (T3). Thyroid cells are the only cells in the body which can absorb iodine. These cells combine iodine and the amino acid tyrosine to make T3 and T4. T3 and T4 are then released into the blood stream and transported throughout the body where they control metabolism (conversion of oxygen and calories to energy). Every cell in the body depends upon thyroid hormones for regulation of metabolism. The normal thyroid gland produces about 80% T4 and about 20% T3. However, T3 possesses about four times the hormone "strength" as T4.

The pituitary gland (a small gland the size of a peanut at the base of the brain) controls the thyroid gland. When the thyroid hormones levels (T3 & T4) drop too low, the pituitary gland produces Thyroid stimulating hormone (TSH) which stimulates the thyroid gland to produce more hormones. Under the influence of TSH, the thyroid will manufacture and secrete T3 and T4 thereby raising their levels in the blood. The pituitary senses this and responds by decreasing TSH production. Imagine the thyroid gland as a furnace and the pituitary gland as the thermostat. Thyroid hormones are like heat. When the heat hits a certain level, the turns thermostat turns off. As the room cools (the thyroid hormone levels drop), the thermostat turns back on (TSH increases) and the furnace produces more heat (thyroid hormones).

The pituitary gland itself is regulated by another gland, known as the hypothalamus. The hypothalamus is part of the brain and produces TSH releasing hormone (TRH) which tells the pituitary gland to stimulate the thyroid gland (release TSH). One might imagine the hypothalamus as the person who regulates the thermostat since it tells the pituitary gland at what level the thyroid should be set.

The thyroid gland, a part of the endocrine (hormone) system, plays a major role in regulating the body's metabolism.

Hypothyroidism is a decreased activity of the thyroid gland which may affect all body functions. The metabolism rate slows causing mental and physical sluggishness. Hypothyroidism can be caused by a thyroid problem (primary), or by the malfunction of the pituitary gland or hypothalamus (secondary**).**

THYROID-STIMULATING HORMONE: When the level of thyroid hormones (T3 & T4) drops too low, the pituitary gland produces Thyroid stimulating hormone (TSH) which stimulates the thyroid gland to produce more hormones.

TITRATING MEDICATION: Continuously measure and adjust the balance of a drug dosage.

TRAUMATIC STRESS: One or more terrifying events in which grave physical harm occurred or was threatened. This stressor may involve serious physical injury, someone's actual death or a threat to the patient's or someone else's life.

TREPIDATION: A term meaning, in general, the fear or trembling. (from Lat. *trepidus*, "anxious")

TSH: See Thyroid Stimulating Hormone.

2A6: An enzyme pathway the body uses to metabolize substances.

2B6: An enzyme pathway the body uses to metabolize substances.

2E1: An enzyme pathway the body uses to metabolize substances.

UGT1A1: This gene encodes an enzyme of a pathway that transforms small molecules, such as steroids, excreted bile, hormones and drugs into water-soluble, excretable substances that have been metabolized.

Lack of UGT1A1 in a newborn's liver is the major cause of jaundice. This jaundice is generally caused by the natural breakdown of fetal blood cells which produces bilirubin that cannot be cleared if UGT1A1 is expressed at low levels or is absent. This type of jaundice can remedied by UV light exposure.

UGT1A3, UGT1A4, UGTIA6, UTGIA9: Human genes used in metabolizing substances in the body. Each gene encodes an enzyme of a pathway that transforms small molecules, such as steroids, excreted bile, hormones and drugs, into water-soluble, excretable substances that have been metabolized.

UGT2B15: A human gene. The UGTs are of major importance in the joining and subsequent elimination of potentially toxic compounds.

UGT2B7: (UDP-Glucuronosyltransferase-2B7) is a phase II metabolism enzyme found to be active in the liver, kidneys, cells of the lower gastrointestinal tract and has also been reported in the brain.UGT2B7 is the major enzyme for the metabolism of morphine.

UNDENATURED: Not having its nature or structure changed; in a natural state not changed in any way.

VAGUS: The vagus nerve, or cranial nerve X, is a part of the autonomic nervous system, which controls functions of the body not under voluntary control, such as heart rate and digestion. The vagus nerve is the only nerve that starts in the brain stem and extends down below the head, to the neck, chest and abdomen.

The medieval Latin word vagus means literally "wandering" (the words vagrant, *vagabond*, and vague come from the same root).

VASOCONSTRICTION: The narrowing of the blood vessels resulting from contraction of the vessel muscular walls. When blood vessels constrict, the flow of blood is restricted or slowed. Factors causing vasoconstriction are called vasoconstrictor, also vasopressors or simply pressors. Vasoconstriction usually results in increased blood pressure. Vasoconstriction may be slight or severe. Vasoconstriction in the penis can disable males from maintaining an erection (erectile dysfunction). It may result from disease, medication or psychological conditions. Medications that cause vasoconstriction include antihistamines, decongestants, methylphenidate (commonly used for ADHD), cough and cold combinations, pseudoephedrine and caffeine.

VASOPRESSIN SECRETION: Arginine vasopressin (AVP), also known as vasopressin, argipressin or antidiuretic hormone (ADH) A hormone found in most mammals, including humans. Primarily increases water re-absorption in the kidneys.

VITAMIN: One of approximately fifteen organic substances essential in small quantities for life and health. Most vitamins cannot be manufactured by the body thus need to be supplied in the diet.

WHEY ISOLATE PROTEIN: Isolate means to separate (a substance) in pure form from a combined mixture. Whey is the watery part of milk that separates from the curd, as in the process of making cheese. What is whey protein? A pure, natural, high quality protein from cow's milk; a rich source of the essential amino acids needed on a daily basis by the body. Its purest form, whey protein isolate, contains little to no fat, lactose or cholesterol.

WITHDRAWAL SIDE EFFECTS: The reactions that occur in your body when you withdraw the use of a drug.

WILLY NILLY: 1. Whether desired or not: *After her boss fell sick, she willy-nilly found herself directing the project.* 2. Being or occurring in a disordered or haphazard fashion: W*illy-nilly zoning laws.*

2A6: An enzyme pathway the body uses to metabolize substances.

2B6: An enzyme pathway the body uses to metabolize substances.

2E1: An enzyme pathway the body uses to metabolize substances.

7 RATING: A rating on how you are doing noted in your journal on The Road Back Program. A 7-10 rating is a rating that you are doing well. You are rating how you feel, your energy, appetite, mood and exercise.

REFERENCES

Ambrosone, C. B., Freudenheim J. L., et al. (1999). "*Manganese superoxide dismutase (MnSOD) genetic polymorphisms, dietary antioxidants, and risk of breast cancer.*" Cancer Res 59(3): 602-6.

Amores-Sanchez, MI, Medina, MA., *Glutamine, as a precursor of glutathione, and oxidative stress.* Mol Genet Metab 1999;67:100-5.

Aynacioglu, A.S., et al. *Frequency of cytochrome P450 CYP2C9 variants in a Turkish population and functional relevance for phenytoin.* Br J Clin Pharmacol 1999; 48(3):409-415

Bailey, L.B., Gregory, J.F., (1999)."*Polymorphisms of methylenetetrahydrofolate reductase and other enzymes: metabolic significance, risks and impact on folate requirement.*" J Nutr 129(5): 919-22

Bailey, L.B., Gregory, J.F., (1999). "*Folate metabolism and requirements.*" J Nutr 129(4): 779-82

Basile, V.S., Masellis, M., Potkin, S.G., Kennedy, J.L., *Pharmacogenomics in schizophrenia: the quest for individualized therapy.* Hum Mol Genet. 2002 Oct 1;11(20):2517-30

Bertilsson, L., et al (1993) *Molecular basis for rational megaprescribing in ultrarapid hydroxylators of debrisoquine.* Lancet 341:63

Blaisdell, J., Mohrenweiser, H., Jackson, Ferguson, J., Coulter, S., Chanas, S., Chanas, B., Xi, T., Ghanayem, B., Goldstein, J.A. *Identification and functional characterization of new potentially defective alleles of human CYP2C19. Pharmacogenetics.* 2002 Dec;12(9):703-11.

Borgstahl, G. E., H. E. Parge, et al. (1996). *"Human mitochondrial manganese superoxide dismutase polymorphic variant Ile58Thr reduces activity by destabilizing the tetrameric interface."* Biochemistry 35(14): 4287-97.

Bosron, W.F., Ting-Kai, L., (1986). *"Genetic polymorphism of human liver alcohol and aldehyde dehydrogenases, and their relationship to alcohol metabolism and alcoholism."* Hepatology 6(3): 502 - 510

Bradford, L.D., *CYP2D6 allele frequency in European Caucasians, Asians, Africans and their descendants.* Pharmacogenomics. 2002 Mar;3 (2):229-43.

Brockmoller, J., et.al. *Pharmacogenetic diagnosis of cytochrome P450 polymorphisms in clinical drug development and in drug treatment.* Pharmacogenetics. 2000:1:125-51.

Bunin, AIa, Filina, A.A., Erchev, V.P., *A glutathione deficiency in open-angle glaucoma and the approaches to its correction.* Vestn Oftalmol 1992;108:13-5 [in Russian].

Cascinu, S., Cordella, L., Del Ferro, E., et al. *Neuroprotective effect of reduced glutathione on cisplatin-based chemotherapy in advanced gastric cancer: a randomized double-blind placebo-controlled trial.* J Clin Oncol 1995;13:26-32.

Ceriello, A., Giugliano, D., Quatraro, A., Lefebvre, P.J., *Anti-oxidants show an anti-hypertensive effect in diabetic and hypertensive subjects.* Clin Sci 1991;81:739-42.

Chang, T.K., et al. *Enhanced cyclophosphamide and ifosfamide activation in primary human hepatocyte cultures: response to cytochrome P-450 inducers and autoinduction by oxazaphosphorines.* Cancer Res 1997; 57(10):1946-54.

Chango, A., Boisson, F., et al. (2000*). "The effect of 677C-->T and 1298A-->C mutations on plasma homocysteine and 5,10-methylenetetrahydrofolate reductase activity in healthy subjects."* Br J Nutr 83(6): 593-6.

Cheng, T., Zhu, Z., et al. (2001). *"Effects of multinutrient supplementation on antioxidant defense systems in healthy human beings."* J Nutr Biochem 12(7): 388-395.

Chida, M., Yokoi, T., Fukui, T., Kinoshita, M., Yokota, J., Kamataki, T., *Detection of three genetic polymorphisms in the 5'-flanking region and intron 1 of human CYP1A2 in the Japanese population.* Jpn J Cancer Res. 1999 Sep;90(9):899-902

Chistyakov, D. A., Savost'anov, et al. (2001). *"Polymorphisms in the Mn-SOD and EC-SOD genes and their relationship to diabetic neuropathy in type 1 diabetes mellitus."* BMC Med Genet 2(1): 4.

Cosma, G., Crofts, F., et al. (1993). *"Relationship between genotype and function of the human CYP1A1 gene."* J Toxicol Environ Health 40(2-3): 309-16.

Cozza, K.L., Armstrong, S.C., Oesterheld, J.R., *Drug Interaction principles for Medical Practice.* American Psychiatric Publishing Inc. (2003)

Crabb, D. W., Edenberg, H. J., et al. (1989). *"Genotypes for aldehyde dehydrogenase deficiency and alcohol sensitivity. The inactive ALDH2(2) allele is dominant."* J Clin Invest 83(1): 314-6.

Crofts, F., Taioli, E., et al. (1994). *"Functional significance of different human CYP1A1 genotypes."* Carcinogenesis 15(12): 2961-3.

Cronin, K. A., Krebs-Smith, S. M., Feuer, E. J., Troiano, R. P., Ballard-Barbash, R., (2001 May). *"Evaluating the impact of population changes in diet, physical activity, and weight status on population risk for colon cancer (United States)".* Cancer Causes Control 12(4):305-16.

Dalhoff K, Ranek L, Mantoni M, Poulsen HE. *Glutathione treatment of hepatocellular carcinoma.* Liver 1992;12:341-3.

Dekou, V., Whincup, P., et al. (2001). *"The effect of the C677T and A1298C polymorphisms in the methylenetetrahydrofolate reductase gene on homocysteine levels in elderly men and women from the British regional heart study."* Atherosclerosis 154(3): 659-66.

De Morais, S.M., Wilkinson, G.R., Blaisdell, J., Nakamura, K., Meyer, U.A., Goldstein, J. *The major genetic defect responsible for the polymorphism of S-mephenytoin metabolism in humans.* J Biol Chem. 1994 Jun 3;269(22):15419-22

De Morais, S.M., Wilkinson, G.R., Blaisdell, J., Meyer, U.A., Nakamura, K., Goldstein, J.A. *Identification of a new genetic defect responsible for the polymorphism of (S)-mephenytoin metabolism in Japanese.* Mol Pharmacol. 1994 Oct;46(4):594-8

Department of Health, London; Stationary Office (2000). *Committee on Medical Aspects of Food and Nutrition Policy. Folic acid and the prevention of disease.*

Donnerstag,,B., Ohlenschläger, Cinatl, J., et al. *Reduced glutathione and S-acetylglutathione as selective apoptosis-inducing agents in cancer therapy.* Cancer Lett 1996;110:63-70.

Eap, C.B., Bender, S., Sirot, E.J., Cucchia, G., Jonzier-Perey, M., Baumann, P., Allorge, D., Broly, F., *Nonresponse to clozapine and ultrarapid CYP1A2 activity: clinical data and analysis of CYP1A2 gene.* Clin Psychopharmacol. 2004 Apr;24(2):214-9

Aklillu, Eleni, Carrillo, Juan Antonio, Makonnen, Eyasu, Hellman, Karin, Pitarque, Marià, Bertilsson, Ingelman-Sundberg, Leif and Magnus *Genetic Polymorphism of CYP1A2 in Ethiopians Affecting Induction and Expression: Characterization of Novel Haplotypes with Single-Nucleotide Polymorphisms in Intron 1.* 2003 Mol Pharmacol 64:659-669.

Evans, William E. and McLeod, Howard L. *Pharmacogenomics — Drug Disposition, Drug Targets, and Side Effects.* New England Journal of Medicine 2003; 348:538-549.

Faber, M.S., Fuhr, U., *Time response of cytochrome P450 1A2 activity on cessation of heavy smoking.* Clin Pharmacol Ther. 2004 Aug;76(2):178-84.

Favilli, F., Marraccini, P., Iantomasis, T., Vincenzini, M.T., *Effect of orally administered glutathione on glutathione levels in some organs of rats: role of specific transporters.* Br J Nutr 1997;78:293-300.

Fennell, T. R., MacNeela, J. P., et al. (2000). *"Hemoglobin adducts from acrylonitrile and ethylene oxide in cigarette smokers: effects of glutathione S-transferase T1-null and M1-null genotypes."* Cancer Epidemiol Biomarkers Prev 9(7): 705-12.

Ferguson, R.J., De Morais, Benhamou, S.M., Benhamou, Bouchardy, S., Bouchardy, C., Blaisdell, J., Ibeanu, G., Wilkinson, G.R., Sarich, T.C., Wright, J.M., Dayer, P., Goldstein, J.A. *A new genetic defect in human CYP2C19: mutation of the initiation codon is responsible for poor metabolism of S-mephenytoin.* J Pharmacol Exp Ther. 1998 Jan;284(1):356-61.

Flagg, E.W., Coates, R.J., Jones, D.P., et al. *Dietary glutathione intake and the risk of oral and pharyngeal cancer.* Am J Epidemiol 1994;139:453-65.

Fohr I.O., Prinz-Lnagenohl, R., et al. (2002). *"10-Methyleneterahydrofolate reductase genotype determines the plasma homocysteine-lowering effect of supplementation with 5-methyltetrahydrofolate or folic acid in healthy young women."* American Journal of Clinical Nutrition 75: 275 - 82

Fontana, R. J., Lown, K. S., et al. (1999). *"Effects of a chargrilled meat diet on expression of CYP3A, CYP1A, and P- glycoprotein levels in healthy volunteers."* Gastroenterology 117(1): 89-98.

Fowke, J.H., Longcope, C., Hebert, J.R., (2000*)* *"Brassica Vegetable Consumption Shifts Estrogen Metabolism in Healthy Postmenopausal Women."* Cancer Epidemiol Biomarkers Prev 9(8):773-779.

Gao, X., Albena T., Dinkova-Kostova, P., Talalay (2001). *"Powerful and prolonged protection of human retinal pigment epithelial cells, keratino-cytes, and mouse leukemia cells against oxidative damage: The indirect antioxidant effects of sulforaphane."* PNAS 98(26): 15221 - 15226.

Garcia-Giralt, E., Perdereau, B., Brixy, F., et al. *Preliminary study of glutathione, L-cysteine and anthocyans (Recancostat Compositum™) in metastatic colorectal carcinoma with malnutrition.* Seventh International Congress on Anti-Cancer Treatment, February 3-6, 1996, Paris, France.

Getahun, S.M., Chung, F.L., (1999). *"Conversion of glucosinolates to isothiocyanates in humans after ingestion of cooked watercress."* Cancer Epidemiology Biomarkers Preview 8(5): 447 - 451.

Giovannucci, E., (1999). *"Nutritional factors in human cancers."* Adv Exp Med Biol 472: 29-42.

Giovannucci, E., Stampfer, M.J., et al. (1998). *"Multivitamin use, folate, and colon cancer in women in the Nurses' Health Study."* Annals of Internal Medicine 129: 517 – 524

Goldstein, J.A., Ishizaki, T., Chiba, K., De Morais, S.M., Bell, D., Krahn, P.M., Evans, D.A. *Frequencies of the defective CYP2C19 alleles responsi-ble for the mephenytoin poor metabolizer phenotype in various Oriental, Caucasian, Saudi Arabian and American black populations.* Pharmacoge-netics 1997, 7: 59-64.

Granfors, M.T., Backman, J.T., Neuvonen, M., Neuvonen, P.J., *Ciproflox-acin greatly increases concentrations and hypotensive effect of tizanidine by inhibiting its cytochrome P450 1A2-mediated presystemic metabolism.* Clin Pharmacol Ther. 2004 Dec;76(6):598-606

Guttmacher, Alan E. and Collins, Francis S. *Genomic Medicine — A Primer.* New England Journal of Medicine 2002; 347:1512-1520.

Guyonnet, D., Belloir, C., Suschetet, M., Siess, M.H., Le Bon, A.M., (2001) *Antimutagenic activity of organosulfur compounds from Allium is associated with phase II enzyme induction.* Mut Res 496(1-2)135-142

Hagen, T.M., Wierzbicka, G.T., Sillau, A.H., et al. *Fate of dietary glutathione: disposition in the gastrointestinal tract.* Am J Physiol 1990;259(4Pt1):G530-5.

Hamdy, S.I., Hiratsuka, M., Narahara, K., Endo, N., El-Enany, M., Moursi, N., Ahmed, M.S., Mizugaki, M., *Genotyping of four genetic polymorphisms in the CYP1A2 gene in the Egyptian population.* Br J Clin Pharmacol. 2003 Mar;55(3):321-4

Hamman, M.A., Thompson, G.A., Hall, S.D., *Regioselective and stereoselective metabolism of ibuprofen by human cytochrome P450 2C.* Biochem Pharmacol 1997; 54(1):33-41.

Harada, S., Agarwal, D. P., et al. (2001). *"Metabolic and ethnic determinants of alcohol drinking habits and vulnerability to alcohol-related disorder."* Alcohol Clin Exp Res 25(5 Suppl ISBRA): 71S-75S.

Heim, M. and Meyer, U.A., *Genotyping of poor metabolisers of debrisoquine by allele-specific PCR amplification.* Lancet 1990; 336:529-532.

Hibbeln, J.R., Umhau, J.C., Linnoila, M., et al. *A replication study of violent and nonviolent subjects: cerebrospinal fluid metabolites of serotonin and dopamine are predicted by plasma essential fatty acids.* Biol Psychiatry 1998;44:243-9.

Higashi, M.K., Veenstra, D.L., Kondo, L.M., Wittkowsky, A.K., Srinouanprachanh, S.L., Farin, F.M., Rettie, A.E., *Association between CYP2C9 genetic variants and anticoagulation-related outcomes during warfarin therapy.* JAMA. 2002 Apr 3;287(13):1690-8.

Ho, P.C., et al. *Influence of CYP2C9 genotypes on the formation of a hepatotoxic metabolite of valproic acid in human liver microsomes.* Pharmacogenomics J 2003; 3(6):335-42.

Hong, C.C., Tang, B.K., Hammond, G.L., Tritchler, D., Yaffe, M., Boyd, N.F., *Cytochrome P450 1A2 (CYP1A2) activity and risk factors for breast cancer: a cross-sectional study.* Breast Cancer Res. 2004;6(4):R352-65. Epub 2004 May 07

Hunjan, M.K., Evered, D.F. *Absorption of glutathione from the gastrointestinal tract.* Biochim Biophys Acta 1985;815:184-8.

Ibeanu, G.C., Blaisdell, J., Ghanayem, B.I., Beyeler, C., Benhamou, S., Bouchardy, C., Wilkinson, G.R., Dayer, P., Daly, A.K., Goldstein, J.A. *An additional defective allele, CYP2C19*5, contributes to the S-mephenytoin poor metabolizer phenotype in Caucasians.* Pharmacogenetics. 1998 Apr;8(2):129-35.

Ibeanu, G.C., Goldstein, J.A., Meyer, U., Benhamou, S., Bouchardy, C., Dayer ,P., Ghanayem, B.I., Blaisdell, J. *Identification of new human CYP2C19 alleles (CYP2C19*6 and CYP2C19*2B) in a Caucasian poor metabolizer of mephenytoin.* J Pharmacol Exp Ther. 1998 Sep;286(3):1490-5.

Inoue, K., Asao, T., et al. (2000*). "Ethnic-related differences in the frequency distribution of genetic polymorphisms in the CYP1A1 and CYP1B1 genes in Japanese and Caucasian populations."* Xenobiotica 30(3): 285-95.1.

Jacques, P. F., Bostom, A. G., et al. (1996). *"Relation between folate status, a common mutation in methylenetetrahydrofolate reductase, and plasma homocysteine concentrations."* Circulation 93(1): 7-9.

Joffe, H.V., Johnson, X.R., Longtine, J., Kucher, N. and Goldhaber, S.Z. *Warfarin dosing and Cytochrome P450 2C9 polymorphisms.* Thromb Haemost; 2004 Jun;91(6):1123-8

Johnston, C.S., Meyer, C.G., Srilakshmi, J.C., *Vitamin C elevates red blood cell glutathione in healthy adults.* Am J Clin Nutr 1993;58:103-5.

Jones, D.P., Coates, R.J., Flagg, E.W., et al. *Glutathione in foods listed in the National Cancer Institute's Health Habits and History Food Frequency Questionnaire.* Nutr Cancer 1995;17:57–75.

Julius, M., Lang, C., Gleiberman, L., et al. *Glutathione and morbidity in a community-based sample of elderly.* J Clin Epidemiol 1994;47:1021-6.

Kalow, W. and Grant, D.M., *Pharmacogenetics - The metabolic and molecular bases of inherited disease.* 1995. Scriver CR, et al, eds. New York: McGraw-Hill, Inc., 293-326

Kang, Z. C., Tsai, S. J., et al. (1999). *"Quercetin inhibits benzo[a]pyrene-induced DNA adducts in human Hep G2 cells by altering cytochrome P-450 1A1 gene expression."* Nutr Cancer 35(2): 175-9.

Kirchheiner, J., Brockmoller, J. *Clinical consequences of cytochrome P450 2C9 polymorphisms.* Clin Pharmacol Ther. 2005 Jan;77(1):1-16.

Kirchheiner, J., Brosen, K., Dahl, M.L., et al.: *CYP2D6 and CYP2C19 genotype-based dose recommendations for antidepressants: a first step towards subpopulation-specific dosages.* Acta Psych Scand 2001 Sept;104(3):173-192.

Kirchheiner, J., Tsahuridu, M., Jabrane, W., Roots, I., Brockmoller, J. *The CYP2C9 polymorphism: from enzyme kinetics to clinical dose recommendations.* Personalized Med 2004 1(1) 63-84

Kirchheiner, J., Nickchen, K., Bauer, M., Wong, M.L., Licinio, J., Roots, I., Brockmoller, J. *Pharmacogenetics of antidepressants and antipsychotics: the contribution of allelic variations to the phenotype of drug response.* Mol Psychiatry. 2004 May;9 (5):442-73.

Kirchheiner, J., et al. *Pharmacogenetics of antidepressants and antipsychotics: the contribution of allelic variations to the phenotype of drug response.* Molecular Psychiatry 2004 9, 442-473

Lam, Y.W.F., Gaedigk, A., Ereshefsy, L., et al: *CYP2D6 inhibition by selective serotonin reuptake inhibitors: analysis of achievable steady-state plasma concentrations and the effect of ultrarapid metabolism at CYP2D6.* Pharmacotherapy 2002;22:1001-1006.

Lampe, J.W., Chen C., et al. (2000). *"Modulation of human glutathione S-transferases by botanically defined vegetable diets."* Cancer Epidemiology Biomarkers Preview 9(8):787-93.

Landi, S., (2000). *"Mammalian class theta GST and differential susceptibility to carcinogens: a review."* Mutat Res 463(3): 247-83.

Lanza, E; Schatzkin, A., Daston, C., Corle, D., Freedman, L., Ballard-Barbash, R., Caan, B., Lance, P., Marshall, J., Iber, F., Shike, M., Weissfeld, J., Slattery, M., Paskett, E., Mateski, D., Albert, P., and the PPT Study Group (2001). *"Implementation of a 4-y, high-fiber, high-fruit-and-vegetable, low-fat dietary intervention: results of dietary changes in the Polyp Prevention Trial 1, 2"* Am J Clin Nutr 74:387-401

Lenzi, A., Picardo, M., Gandini, L., et al. *Glutathione treatment of dyspermia: effect on the lipoperoxidation process.* Hum Reprod 1994;9:2044-50.

Lenzi, A., Culasso, F., Gandini, L., et al. *Placebo-controlled, double-blind, cross-over trial of glutathione therapy in male infertility.* Hum Reprod 1993;8:1657-62.

Lewis, D.F., Lake, B.G., Dickins, M., *Substrates of human cytochromes P450 from families CYP1 and CYP2: analysis of enzyme selectivity and metabolism.* Drug Metabol Drug Interact. 2004;20(3):111-42.

Lin, H.J., Probst-Hensch, N.M., Louie, A.D., Kau, I.H., Witte, J.S., Ingles, S.A., Frankl, H.D., Lee, E.R., Haile, R.W., (1998 Aug). *"Glutathione transferase null genotype, broccoli, and lower prevalence of colorectal adenomas."* Cancer Epidemiol Biomarkers Prev 7(8):647-52.

Linder, M.W., Prough, R.A., Valdes, R. Jr. Pharmacogenetics: *a laboratory tool for optimizing therapeutic efficiency.* Clin Chem 1997;43:254-66.

Linder, M.W., Valdes, R .Jr. *Pharmacogenetics in the Practice of Laboratory Medicine. Molecular Diagnosis.* 1999;4:365-79.

Linder, M.W., Valdes, R. Jr. *Genetic mechanisms for variability in drug response and toxicity.* J Anal Toxicol 2001;25:405-13.

Linder, M.W., Valdes, R. Jr. *Pharmacogenetics in the practice of laboratory medicine.* Mol Diagn 1999;4:365-79.

Linder, M.W., Valdes, R. Jr. *Fundamentals and applications of pharmacogenetics for the clinical laboratory.* Ann Clin Lab Sci 1999;29:140-9.

London, S. J., Yuan, J. M., et al. (2000). *"Isothiocyanates, glutathione S-transferase M1 and T1 polymorphisms, and lung-cancer risk: a prospective study of men in Shanghai, China."* Lancet 356(9231): 724-9.

Lundqvist, E., Johansson, I., Ingelman-Sundberg, M. *Genetic mechanisms for duplication and multiduplication of the human CYP2D6 gene and methods for detection of duplicated CYP2D6 genes.* Gene 1999 Jan 21;226(2):327-338.

Lutz, W. K., *"Carcinogens in the diet vs overnutrition. Individual dietary habits, malnutrition, and genetic susceptibility modify carcinogenic potency and cancer risk."* Mutation Research (1999) 443: 251-258

Marez, D., Legrand, M., Sabbagh, N., Guidice, J.M., Spire, C., Lafitte, J.J., Meyer, U.A., Broly, F. *Polymorphism of the cytochrome P450 CYP2D6 gene in a European population: characterization of 48 mutations and 53 alleles, their frequencies and evolution.* Pharmacogenetics. 1997 Jun;7(3):193-202.

Michaud, D.S., Spiegelman, D., et al.(1999). *"Fruit and vegetable intake and incidence of bladder cancer in a male prospective cohort."* J Natl Cancer Inst 91(7): 605-13.

Miller, M.C. 3rd, Mohrenweiser, H.W., Bell, D.A. (2001) *"Genetic variability in susceptibility and response to toxicants."* Toxicol Lett 120(1-3):269-80

Miners, J. *CYP2C9 polymorphism: impact on tolbutamide pharmacokinetics and response.* Pharmacogenetics 2002; 12(2):91-2.

Molloy, J., Martin, J.F., Baskerville, P.A., et al. *S-nitrosoglutathione reduces the rate of embolization in humans. Circulation* 1998;98:1372-5.

Nakajima, M., Yokoi, T., Mizutani, M., Kinoshita, M., Funayama, M., Kamataki, T. *Genetic polymorphism in the 5'-flanking region of human CYP1A2 gene: effect on the CYP1A2 inducibility in humans.* J Biochem (Tokyo). 1999 Apr;125(4):803-8

Nemets, B., Stahl, Z., Belmaker,R.H. *Addition of omega-3 fatty acid to maintenance medication treatment for recurrent unipolar depressive disorder.* Am J Psychiatry 2002;159:477–9.

Nijhoff, W.A., Mulder, T.P., et al. (1995*). "Effects of consumption of Brussels sprouts on plasma and urinary glutathione S-transferase class-alpha and -pi in humans."* Carcinogenesis 16(4): 955-7.

Parke, D.V. (1999). *"Antioxidants and disease prevention: mechanisms of action".* Antioxidants in Human Health. CABI Publishing.

Perera, F. P. and Weinstein, I. B. (2000). *"Molecular epidemiology: recent advances and future directions."* Carcinogenesis 21(3): 517-24.

Peyvandi, F., Spreafico, M., Siboni, S.M., Moia, M. and Mannucci, P.M. *CYP2C9 genotypes and dose requirements during the induction phase of oral anticoagulation therapy.* Clinical Pharmacology and Therapeutics 2004; 75(3):198-203

Regier, D.A., Narrow, W.E., Rae, D.S., et al. *The de facto US mental and addictive disorders service system. Epidemiologic Catchment Area prospective 1-year prevalence rates of disorders and services.* Arch Gen Psychiatry 1993;50:85–94.

Rozen, R. (2000). *"Genetic modulation of homocysteinemia."* Semin Thromb Hemost 26(3): 255-61.

Rettie, A.E., et al. *Impaired (S)-warfarin metabolism catalysed by the R144C allelic variant of CYP2C9.* Pharmacogenetics 1994; 4(1):39-42.

Sachse, C., Brockmoller, J., Bauer, S., Roots, I. *Functional significance of a C-->A polymorphism in intron 1 of the cytochrome P450 CYP1A2 gene tested with caffeine.* Br J Clin Pharmacol. 1999 Apr;47(4):445-9

Sandhu, M.S., White, I.R., McPherson, K. (2001). *"Systematic review of the prospective cohort studies on meat consumption and colorectal cancer risk: a meta-analytical approach."* Cancer Epidemiol Biomarkers Prev 10(5): 439-46

Schuppe, H.C., Wieneke, P., Donat, S., Fritsche, E., Kohn, F.M., Abel, J. (2000). *"Xenobiotic metabolism, genetic polymorphisms and male infertility."* Andrologia 32(4-5): 255-62

Scordo, M.G., et al. *Genetic polymorphism of cytochrome P450 2C9 in a Caucasian and a black African population.* Br J Clin Pharmacol 2001; 52(4):447-450.

Sechi, G., Deledda, M.G., Bua, G., et al. *Reduced intravenous glutathione in the treatment of early Parkinson's disease.* Prog Neuropsychopharmacol Biol Psychiatry 1996;20:1159-70.

Sen, C.K. *Nutritional biochemistry of cellular glutathione.* Nutr Biochem 1997;8:660-72.

Sinha, R., Chow, W.H., Kulldorff, M., Denobile, J., Butler, J., Garcia-Closas, M., Weil, R., Hoover, R.N., Rothman, N. (1999). *"Well-done, grilled red meat increases the risk of colorectal adenomas."* Cancer Res 59(17): 4320-4

Smith, T.J., Yang, C.S. (2000). *"Effect of organosulfur compounds from garlic and cruciferous vegetables on drug metabolism enzymes."* Drug Metabol Drug Interact 17(1-4):23-49

Solus, J.F., Arietta, B.J., Harris, J.R., Sexton, D.P., Steward, J.Q., McMunn, C., Ihrie, P., Mehall, J.M., Edwards, T.L., Dawson, E.P. *Genetic variation in eleven phase I drug metabolism genes in an ethnically diverse population.* Pharmacogenomics. 2004 Oct;5(7):895-931.

Spiteri, M. A., Bianco, A., et al. (2000). *"Polymorphisms at the glutathione S-transferase, GSTP1 locus: a novel mechanism for susceptibility and development of atopic airway inflammation."* Allergy 55(Suppl 61): 15-20.

Steen, V.M., et al. *Detection of the poor metabolizer-associated CYP2D6(D) gene deletion by long-PCR technology.* Pharmacogenetics 1995; 5:215-223.

Steinkellner, H., Rabot, S., Freywald, C., Nobis, E., Scharf, G., Chabi-covsky, M., Knasmuller, S., Kassie, F. (2001). *"Effects of cruciferous vegetables and their constituents on drug metabolizing enzymes involved in the bioactivation of DNA-reactive dietary carcinogens."* Mutat Res 480-481: 285-97

Stoll, A.L., Severus, W.E., Freeman, M.P., et al. *Omega 3 fatty acids in bipolar disorder: a preliminary double-blind, placebo-controlled trial.* Arch Gen Psychiatry 1999;56:407–12.

Strange, R. C., Spiteri, M. A., et al. (2001). *"Glutathione-S-transferase family of enzymes."* Mutat Res 482(1-2): 21-6.

Smyth, J.F., Bowman, A., Perren, T., et al. *Glutathione reduces the toxicity and improves quality of life of women diagnosed with ovarian cancer treated with cisplatin: results of a double-blind, randomised trial. Ann Oncol* 1997;8:569-73.

Takahashi, H., Echizen, H. *Pharmacogenetics of warfarin elimination and its clinical implications.* Clin Pharmacokinet 2001; 40(8):587-603.

Takeshita, T. and Morimoto, K. (2000). *"Accumulation of hemoglobin-associated acetaldehyde with habitual alcohol drinking in the atypical ALDH2 genotype."* Alcohol Clin Exp Res 24(1): 1-7.

Testa, B., Mesolella, M., Testa, D. *Glutathione in the upper respiratory tract. Ann Otol Rhinol Laryngol* 1995;104:117-9.

Trickler, D., Shklar, G., Schwartz, J. *Inhibition of oral carcinogenesis by glutathione. Nutr Cancer* 1993;20:139-44.

Ueland, P. M., Hustad, S., et al. (2001). *"Biological and clinical implications of the MTHFR C677T polymorphism."* Trends Pharmacol Sci 22(4): 195-201.

Vakevainen, S., Tillonen, J., Agarwal, D.P., Srivastava, N., Salaspuro, M. (2000). *"High salivary acetaldehyde after a moderate dose of alcohol in*

ALDH2-deficient subjects: strong evidence for the local carcinogenic action of acetaldehyde. " Alcohol Clin Exp Res 22(4): 195-201

Van der Weide, J. and Steijns, L.S.W. *Cytochrome P450 enzyme system: genetic polymorphisms and impact on clinical pharmacology.* Ann Clin Biochem 1999; 36:722-729.

Van Iersel, M.L., Verhagen, H., et al. (1999). *"The role of biotransformation in dietary (anti)carcinogenesis."* Mutation Research 443(1-2): 259-70.

Van Landeghem, G. F., Tabatabaie, P., et al. (1999). *"Ethnic variation in the mitochondrial targeting sequence polymorphism of MnSOD."* Hum Hered 49(4): 190-3.

Vendemiale, G., Altomare, E., Trizio, T., et al. *Effects of oral S-adenosyl-L-methionine on hepatic glutathione in patients with liver disease. Scand J Gastroenterol* 1989;24:407-15.

Verhoeff, B. J., Trip, M. D., et al. (1998). *"The effect of a common methyle-netetrahydrofolate reductase mutation on levels of homocysteine, folate, vitamin B12 and on the risk of premature atherosclerosis."* Atherosclerosis 141(1): 161-6.

Wang, S.T., Chen, H.W., Sheen, L.Y., Lii, C.K. *Methionine and cysteine affect glutathione level, glutathione-related enzyme activities and the expression of glutathione S-transferase isozymes in rat hepatocytes. J Nutr* 1997;127:2135-41.

Wang, X., Zuckerman, B., et al. (2002) *"Maternal cigarette smoking, metabolic gene polymorphism, and infant birth weight."* Journal of the American Medical Association 287(2): 195 - 202

Weinshilboum, Richard. *Inheritance and Drug Response* New England Journal of Medicine 2003; 348:529-537

White, A.C., Thannickal, V.J., Fanburg, B.L. *Glutathione deficiency in human disease. J Nutr Biochem* 1994;5:218–26.

Willett, W.C. (1995). *"Diet, nutrition, and avoidable cancer".* Environ Health Perspect 103(Suppl 8): 165-170

Williams, J.A., Martin, F.L., Muir, G.H., Hewer, A., Grover, P.L., Phillips, D.H. (2000). *"Metabolic activation of carcinogens and expression of various cytochromes P450 in human prostate tissue."* Carcinogenesis 21(9): 1683-9.

Witschi, A., Reddy, S., Stofer, B., Lauterburg, B.H. *The systemic availability of oral glutathione. Eur J Clin Pharmacol* 1992;43:667-9.

Wolf ,C.R. and Smith, G. *Pharmacogenetics.* Br Med Bull 1999; 55(2):366-386.

Xiao, Z.S., Goldstein, J.A., Xie, H.G., Blaisdell, J., Wang, W., Jiang, C.H., Yan, F.X., He, N., Huang, S.L., Xu, Z.H., Zhou, H.H. *Differences in the incidence of the CYP2C19 polymorphism affecting the S-mephenytoin phenotype in Chinese Han and Bai populations and identification of a new rare CYP2C19 mutant allele.* J Pharmacol Exp Ther. 1997 Apr;281(1):604-9.

Yamauchi, M., Takeda, K., Sakamoto, K., Searashi, Y., Uetake, S., Kenichi, H., Toda, G. (2001). *"Association of polymorphism in the alcohol dehydrogenase 2 gene with alcohol-induced testicular atrophy."* Alcohol Clin Exp Res 25(Suppl 6): 16-8

Yechiel Levkovitz, Galit Ben-shushan, Hershkovitz, Isaac, Gil-Ad, Shvartsman, Ronen, Weizman, Zick. (2007) Mol Cell Neuroscience. Antidepressants induce cellular insulin resistance by activation of IRS-1 kinases.

Yokoyama, A., Muramatsu, T., Ohmori, T., Yokoyama, T., Okuyama, K., Takahashi, H., Hasegawa, Y., Higuchi, S., Maruyama, K., Shirakura, K., Ishii, H. (1998). *"Alcohol-related cancers and aldehyde dehydrogenase-2 in Japanese alcoholics."* Carcinogenesis 19(8):1383-7

Zackrisson, A.L., Lindblom, B. *Identification of CYP2D6 alleles by single nucleotide polymorphism analysis using pyrosequencing.* Eur J Clin Pharmacol. 2003 Oct;59 (7):521-6.

Zhao, B., Seow, A, Lee, E.J., Poh, W.T., The, M., Eng, P., Wang, Y.T., Tan, W.C., Yu, M.C., Lee, H.P. (2001*). "Dietary isothiocyanates, glutathione S-transferase -M1, -T1 polymorphisms and lung cancer risk among Chinese women in Singapore."* Cancer Epidemiol Biomarkers Prev 10(10): 1063-7

Zusterzeel, P.L., Nelen, W.L., Roelofs, H.M., Peters, W.H., Blom, H.J., Steegers, E.A. (2000). *"Polymorphisms in biotransformation enzymes and the risk for recurrent early pregnancy loss."* Mol Hum Reprod 6(5): 474-8

"Who would have thought, one tiny decision could not only nearly kill you but take 9 months of your life away.

This was what thought would be a painless, ultimately beneficial decision made November 19th 2006.

I decided to quit taking my 2 1/2 mg of Valium. I had been taking it nearly every night at bedtime for the last 3 years. My first BIG MISTAKE! I, in my naivety didn't have the slightest clue that I was totally dependent on the little yellow pill. Who could ever have thought something so small could be so powerful.

Let's just say 2 weeks later I ended up having to dial 911. I was alone, it was nighttime and I thought I was dying. I ended up in the emergency room, the doctors not having a clue what was wrong with me.

I had told the paramedic I had stopped taking my Diazepam. He either didn't think it was important, or didn't tell the doctors in the ER. For 3 hours I was hallucinating and going literally insane all alone in that ER surrounded by a curtain that was breathing and moving.

I thought I had slit my wrists when I looked down and the doctor was trying to take blood. My brain wasn't working properly. Finally I was able to call my husband and he told the attending that 2 weeks prior I had quit taking Valium. I had to convince the doctors to talk to my husband, since I wasn't making much sense anymore. They finally spoke to him.

I still remember the female attending saying" Oh, why didn't she tell us that." Well, try thinking clearly when everyone around you is speaking Russian and the curtains are alive and breathing. Try thinking when the staff are treating you like a common junkie. The doctor quickly gave me a shot of something and my world came back. Literally 10 minutes later they were talking about discharging me and I was calling a taxi.

I though the worst was over. My second BIG MISTAKE.

I went with the ER doctor's advice of reducing my pills by 50 percent every 2 weeks. This took 6 weeks. I extended it to 8 weeks because I didn't feel great. My family doctor sent me to a neurologist who agreed with the reduction. I basically got worse and worse the longer I was off the pills.

I had to go on an emergency Xanax prescription because I had been nominated for an Oscar and wanted to go to the ceremony. Oh ya, didn't I mention this, while all this hell was going on... I got nominated for a Oscar.... Stressful......Oh just a little.

I wanted to go to the ceremony and had been feeling worse since quitting the pills. I went on the Xanax for about a week, made it thru the ceremony, then 5 days later I crashed again. Not as bad as the time before, no 911, no hallucinating, but very scary. I had to go back on the Xanax.

Ok, I was in trouble again. I didn't understand why... what was going on? Why wasn't I better? How could I be getting worse? None of it made sense.

Back with my neurologist, he thought I was feeling bad because I didn't win the Oscar. Dear god, you must be joking... that was it for him. Time for a new doctor. He thought I was under stress, which I was, but wanted to put me on Buspar. I didn't want any more pills. Couldn't anyone understand that, look where pills had gotten me.

My husband and myself spent hours on the Internet looking for help and advice. I was now back on the Valium but didn't feel well. Didn't feel myself anymore. I felt like I was constantly falling into myself. It's hard to describe, but I literally felt like I was imploding. Headaches, breathing problems, depression, anxiety, chest pains you name it I was experiencing it. I was now on over 3 mg a night and still no relief. What was happening, why didn't it all go away and I feel better like my GP and neurologist said it should.

Why was I feeling worse and worse?

Then something happened... Independently, but on the same day, both myself and my husband came across the Road Back on the Internet. Finally, something that made sense, something that actually spoke to me, addressed my problems, acknowledged this was happening and had been happening to thousands and thousands of other poor souls.

Nirvana! I had found my road back.

I called one of the doctors recommenced on the site and went to see her within a week. She spoke my language, she understood, I wasn't invisible. There was hope. This was at the end of March 2007.

I immediately went on the program, the Essential Protein Powder helped immediately. The Body Calm capsules I had to get used to, I was afraid of anything that might have power over the body. I felt I had lost control of. I had to trust the doctor and let go. All the other powders and pills came and I started to feel a bit better. A bit stronger. It wasn't some overnight miracle, it wasn't a flash of lightning. But, it was working.

I realized how dangerous all this had been, I realized the dangers of the drug from the Road Back Web Site, and now I had to come to terms with the fact that I was still taking the evil Valium. The pill I had felt nearly killed me. I was having not only to take every night but increase it.

I finally got to 4 mg per night. Why wasn't I able to stabilize? Why wasn't I getting better quicker. Basically, I had to stabilize before I could start to reduce the Valium. It just wasn't happening. I wasn't stabilizing. Sure, I was feeling better, but I wasn't coming to the place where I could start to reduce.

I made my 3rd BIG MISTAKE!

Through the advice of a friend, I went to see a pharmacological psychologist. The doctor basically told me this all was a sham and I needed to go on multiple drugs. Anxiety pills, antidepressants and god knows what else. She basically told me I wasn't still having problems from the Valium, I was the problem. It couldn't still be from the pill, because I was taking it every night. I had psychological problems and needed to take more pills! Are you kidding me? More pills? I was mentally sick? I was the problem?

I went to see Dr. Shields again, I was a mess. I was now freaked I was going insane. She was wonderful, she hugged me and held me, she said how sorry she was that I had to hear those things. She was disgusted with the psychologist who told me those things.

The psychologist didn't understand withdrawal and obviously wasn't part of the Road Back. The Road Back doctor wanted me to speak to

Jim Harper, the founder of the Road Back. I talked with him the next day. My world changed that day and again 2 days later.

Jim was very gracious and very understanding. He listened and then said he thought he could help. He was going to send me a new herbal product he had been testing. It was made from the Passion Flower plant. A plant?

Great, I'll give it a shot, as long as it doesn't come from a pharmaceutical company. He talked with me for over an hour and made lots of suggestions and just listened. The Passion Flower arrived the next day. I took my first pill that night around 5 pm. That was when I had been having to take a 1/2 mg of Valium.

I hadn't been able to wait until bed time, my brain felt like it was falling out, I had been taking Valium during the day since my visit to the psychologist. She really freaked me out. Now I was anxiety ridden, I was a mess.

The passion flower arrived and I took it at my usual brain falling out time. Something happened! Well, more accurately nothing happened. My brain didn't fall out. I felt normal....The passion flower 100% worked.

It calmed me down without making me feel drugged. It acted as a natural Valium in a way. It completely relieved my withdrawal symptom! My god, a miracle!

Over the next few weeks I tweaked the pill size and amount of times I took it. I had to find the balance. Jim was there for me on the phone or our preferred way, via email the entire time. He wanted to know how I was doing, how my symptoms were and my anxiety levels. I was his lab rat. Oh what a happy rat I was!

For the first time in 6 months I felt like there was hope for me. Hope that I would again be normal, hope that this wasn't going to last forever. Jim gave me that hope back. He saved my life. I know that sounds overly dramatic, but it's true. The road back saved my sanity and my life. I no longer cried every day, I no longer thought every pain would end up with me in the hospital. I was no longer was afraid.

I have been taking the Passion Flower now for a about 2 months. I began to finally stabilize. I could finally start reducing the Valium. The day I was waiting for: 6 months came a few weeks ago. The day I could go to a compounding pharmacy and start reducing the pill I had come to call Satan. The passion flower; now known as Body Calm Supreme, is now available thru TRB Health.

Don't get me wrong. It's not all happy shiny clouds and little new-born kittens. I still have bad times. But that's just it now. They are times. Not full time.

When I first started reducing I got a little over zealous and reduced too much. I slowed down after talking to Jim. Then I reduced every week, again, it was too much for me, and after talking to Jim I am now reducing every 2 weeks. Sure it's slow, sure it will take me the rest of the year. It will take me 8 months not 8 weeks. But you know what, when you feel good again, when you feel hopeful, time doesn't really matter so much.

When you have come so close to the edge, when you have given up all hope, what's a bit of time? What's a few months when you have been given those months back. You can actually live those months out in the real world, not at home shut in and invisible.

I can't stress enough what life is like now. How precious every moment is. How all that really matters is your health and well being. How much love you have in your life can actually save your life.

For months I was angry, I was angry because unless your some crack addict or celebrity drunk, you don't exist. I was angry because I felt invisible. There just wasn't any help out there for me.

Valium isn't a trendy drug, no one cares if you're dependent on it. I was a functioning addict without even knowing it. The film business is so stressful, I took the Valium to relax and be able to slow my mind down so I could sleep. I have had trouble sleeping my entire life. I was an accident waiting to happen. Now, I'll take the Body Calm and the Body CalmSupreme, thank you very much.

Jim listened to me when I needed it most. The Road Back doctor cared for me when I needed it most. My husband stood by me the entire time. My family never judged me. My friends listened and offered their support. I have seen a new way to deal with stress in the future.

You have to realize it's a slow, slow battle. As Jim always says, slow and steady wins the race. You can't forget that even though you feel as if your not getting better quick enough, or you don't even feel you'll ever get better. You will, just follow the plan, stick to the rules, listen to your body.

I'm sure the route I chose to go, the non-multiple drug route cost me time in the end. I'm sure the drugs would have been a quick fix, I probably would have felt better quicker. But that wasn't my way. No more drugs, no more pills. I wanted to do it under my own steam, for better or worse. I didn't want to swap one addiction for another. It's what everyone seems to do. Just take another pill. Not me, no way!

No film is worth this stress. An Oscar nomination doesn't take the pain away. I will manage my stress better in the future. I will take my health more seriously from now on. I will never take any prescription pills again. I will listen to my body. And, I will always listen to Jim." J.O.

9506128R0

Made in the USA
Lexington, KY
03 May 2011